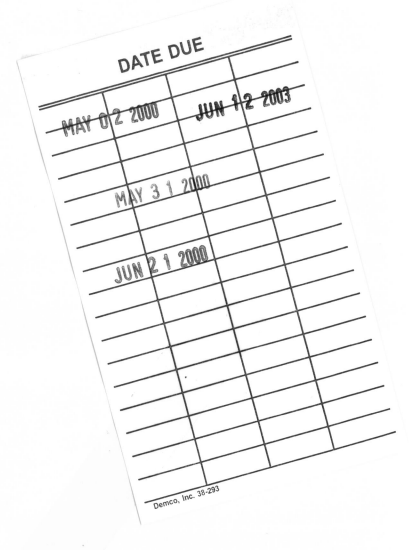

DATE DUE

MAY 0 2 2000		JUN 1 2 2003
	MAY 3 1 2000	
	JUN 2 1 2000	

Demco, Inc. 38-293

STRESS REDUCTION
FOR CAREGIVERS

STRESS REDUCTION FOR CAREGIVERS

Jodi L. Olshevski, M.S.G.
Boston, Massachusetts

Anne D. Katz, Ph.D.
Bob G. Knight, Ph.D.
Andrus Gerontology Center
University of Southern California
Los Angeles, California

with guest author

T. J. McCallum, M.A.
Andrus Gerontology Center
University of Southern California
Los Angeles, California

USA	Publishing Office:	BRUNNER/MAZEL *A member of the Taylor & Francis Group* 325 Chestnut Street Philadelphia, PA 19106 Tel: (215) 625-8900 Fax: (215) 625-2940
	Distribution Center:	BRUNNER/MAZEL *A member of the Taylor & Francis Group* 47 Runway Road, Suite G Levittown, PA 19057 Tel: (215) 269-0400 Fax: (215) 269-0363
UK		BRUNNER/MAZEL *A member of the Taylor & Francis Group* 1 Gunpowder Square London EC4A 3DE Tel: +44 171 583 0490 Fax: +44 171 583 0581

STRESS REDUCTION FOR CAREGIVERS

1 2 3 4 5 6 7 8 9 0

Printed by Braun-Brumfield, Ann Arbor, MI, 1999.
Cover design by Curt Tow.

A CIP catalog record for this book is available from the British Library.
⊚ The paper in this publication meets the requirements of the ANSI Standard Z39.48-1984 (Permanence of Paper).

Library of Congress Cataloging-in-Publication Data

Olshevski, Jodi.
    Stress reduction for caregivers / Jodi Olshevski, Anne Katz, Bob Knight
with guest author T.J. McCallum.
        p.   cm.
    Includes bibliographical references and index.
    ISBN 0-87630-940-6 (alk. paper). -- ISBN 0-87630-941-4 (alk.
paper)
    1. Aged--Home care--Psychological aspects. 2. Alzheimer's
disease--Patients--Home care--Psychological aspects. 3. Senile
dementia--Patients--Home care--Psychological aspects.
    4. Caregivers--Mental health. 5. Stress management. I. Knight,
Bob. II. Olshevski, Jodi. III. Title.
HV1451.K39 1999
155.9′042′08836--dc21   98-55754
                                                                            CIP

ISBN 0-87630-940-6
    0-87630-941-4

CONTENTS

Preface   IX

1

Stress and Coping Models of Caregiving Distress   1

Stress and Coping Models   3
Is Caregiving Stressful Because It Is Hard Work?   6
The Course of Caregiving Distress   7
Stress and Coping Models and the Intervention Presented
   in This Volume   7
Summary   12
References   13

2

Dementia Caregiver Burden and Ethnicity, *T. J. McCallum*   17

Sociocultural Factors and Social Support   18
Cultural Tradition   19
Family Dynamics   20
Case Example   21
The Role of the Church   22
Caregiver Ethnicity and Coping Style   23
Theoretical Explanations   25
Stress Buffering   26
Physiological Research   27
Caregiving and Physiological Stress: A Review of the
   Literature   27
Caregiving and Poor Health Outcomes   29
Summary   30
References   30

3

Stress Level Monitoring   35

Understanding Stress   35
The Cycle of Distress   38
The Use of Monitoring   39
The Daily Stress Rating Form   40
Case Examples   43
Summary   48
References   49

4

Progressive Relaxation and Visualization   51

Progressive Relaxation   51
Visualization   55
Case Examples   56
Summary   62
References   63

5

The Relaxing Events Schedule   65

Caring for Self   65
Pleasant Events Theory   66
Caregiver Stress and Relaxing Events   68
The Relaxing Events Schedule   69
Case Example   76
Summary   79
References   79

6

Stress-Neutral Thoughts   81

Cognitive Restructuring   81
Cognitive Restructuring: Caregivers and Older Adults   84
Worried Thoughts   86
The Thought Tracking Record   87
Reducing Worried Thoughts and Increasing Stress-Neutral
   Thoughts   89
Elements of Self-Change   90
Case Examples   91
Summary   96
References   97

7   **The Effectiveness of the Stress Reduction Technique**   **99**

A Brief Review of the Interventions   **99**
The Effects of Psychoeducational Intervention on
    Self-Reported Distress in Caregivers   **104**
Case Examples   **109**
Summary   **114**
References   **114**

8   **The Context of Stress Reduction: Community Services**
and Resources for Caregivers   **117**

Respite Services and Community-Based Services   **117**
Placement in 24-Hour Care   **123**
Legal Alternatives   **126**
Options After Incapacity   **129**
Medicaid and Medi-Cal   **130**
Psychosocial Interventions   **132**
Summary   **134**
References   **135**

Index   **137**

PREFACE

This approach to understanding and reducing emotional distress in family caregivers of older relatives with dementia was developed over the past 9 years at the Tingstad Older Adult Counseling Center and the Alzheimer's Disease Research Center (a National Institute on Aging [NIA] funded research center, Caleb Finch, principal investigator [PI]) at the University of Southern California (USC) Andrus Gerontology Center. As is the case in any long-term research and development program, a large number of people have contributed to the work that is reported in this volume.

In 1989, I received a grant from the Robert Ellis Simon Foundation which funded the first version of caregiving interventions that eventually developed into the stress reduction training program. In that first year, we worked with caregivers in groups and used an approach that focused on education about dementing illnesses (Alzheimer's disease, vascular dementias, and so forth) and discussed problem-solving strategies as well as use of relaxation training and other stress reduction strategies.

At around the same time, Hortense Tingstad (whose endowment has supported the continued operation of the Tingstad Older Adult Counseling Center) was lending enthusiastic support to the development of stress reduction strategies over lunch in the tearoom at the old Bullock's Wilshire in Los Angeles and during early morning phone calls. Ms. Tingstad had benefitted from a short stress reduction treatment from a psychologist at her health maintenance organization (HMO) during an early phase of caring for her husband.

Also about the same time, stress and coping models began to emerge as the dominant conceptual paradigm for thinking about outcomes of caregiving, including caregivers' emotional distress. Our current thinking about stress and coping models for caregiver distress is outlined in chapter 1. This thinking is influenced largely by Folkman and Lazarus's theoretical models of stress and coping as well as by the work of Leonard Pearlin and of Peter Vitaliano.

In 1989–1990, we received a budget augmentation from the NIA to USC's Alzheimer's Disease Research Center, which was used to fund additional psychoeducational groups for caregivers and to develop manuals and videotapes for problem-solving training and stress reduction training. Both approaches included education about dementia, education about community resources, and sections on using social support wisely. The problem-solving approach follows the strategies outlined in Zarit, Orr, and Zarit's *The Hidden Victims of Alzheimer's Disease: Families Under Stress* (1985). It focuses primarily on teaching caregivers problem-solving skills and behavioral techniques to reduce problems with the care recipient which, in turn, should reduce caregivers' distress. The stress reduction manual contained the elements of the approach described here: relaxation training, scheduling of relaxing events, and cognitive restructuring. As described in chapters 4 and 6, relaxation training and cognitive restructuring are common elements of cognitive behavioral therapy and have been used widely for stress reduction in other populations by, among others, Donald Meichenbaum and Albert Ellis. The relaxing events notion was directly adapted from the pleasant events component of Peter Lewinsohn's behavioral therapy for depression (see chapter 5). These techniques are designed to directly reduce the caregiver's emotional distress. Anne Katz headed up the development of these manuals, with substantial assistance from Jacque Lehn, Marie Liston, Jodi Olshevski, Susan Thurgood, Richard Wurster, Mark Beers, Richard A. Lehn, Richard M. Lehn, and Brad Williams.

From late 1989 through 1992, we were funded by the Alzheimer's Disease Research Program of the California Department of Health Services (the "tax checkoff" monies) to do research on the stress and coping model of caregiving and to compare the problem-solving therapy and stress reduction training approaches. Jodi Olshevski, then a student in the master's degree program in gerontology at USC and Steven Lutzky, then a doctoral student in gerontology at USC, were the key research assistants in that project. At this point, we switched to individual stress reduction training, with most of the training being in the caregivers' homes. The group training sessions in 1989 had not proven to be cost-effective for us because groups were hard to arrange and tended to disband quickly if one or two members became ill, placed their relatives, or took a vacation. We also came to realize that recruiting caregivers who could leave the relative with dementia at home and come to a group every week tended to screen out caregivers of relatives with more severe impairments and caregivers who were more seriously distressed—the very people that we wanted to interview and to help.

At the end of this project, we evaluated the outcomes of the two approaches and also reflected on our experiences with the two types of training. The quantitative evaluation results are summarized in chapter 7. Although this clearly was a small, pilot study, we felt that the results favored stress reduction training. Our trainers unanimously reported that caregivers preferred the stress reduction approach and seemed to find it more helpful.

There were aspects of this version of the training that we felt needed revision and improvement. A key issue was the feeling that we were trying to cover too much material in too short a time and that there was only limited time to follow up with the caregivers to see if they were regularly using the interventions and to identify problems that came up in using these strategies so that they could be individualized for each caregiver's unique situation and personal needs.

We then decided to delete education about dementing illnesses in order to leave more time to focus on the stress reduction interventions. In our evaluations of this pilot project, knowledge about dementia was uncorrelated with distress and did not change much during the training. Our observation was that most caregivers already knew a lot about dementing illnesses. When they did not, it was easy to give them information to read or to refer them to educational events in the community. We also found that, after a certain basic orientation to the illness, more information about dementia is not necessarily helpful in terms of reducing distress.

We also put the information about community resources "outside of" the stress reduction training sessions. The issue here is that this background information is needed by stress reduction trainers so that they can make accurate referrals as needed for caregivers' specific problems. However, it is unnecessary to educate each individual caregiver about the full range of community resources, many of which will not be relevant. Chapter 8 provides an overview of typical community resources for caregiving families. We have tried to make it as general as possible, but services, resources, and laws vary from state to state and often from community to community. As I have argued elsewhere about psychotherapy with older adults (Knight, 1996), it is necessary to understand the context of community services for frail older people, and especially for adults with dementia and their families, in order to perform effective psychological interventions.

These changes produced a version of stress reduction training which essentially is focused entirely on the three change techniques, beginning with teaching caregivers to monitor their stress levels (as described in chapter 3). Monitoring stress is key to understanding the sources of stress and of relaxation and to help the caregiver notice the small, gradual changes that are typical during the training. As described in chapter 3, stress monitoring itself sometimes can reduce perceived stress, especially by disproving the perception that one is stressed to the same extent all of the time.

By focusing on fewer techniques, more time is available to work with the caregivers to be sure that they use the techniques at home and to analyze and solve problems that arise in using the techniques in the individual situation of the specific caregiver. This approach has been used in our project under the direction of Donna Benton at the Alzheimer's Disease Research Center since 1994. As this volume goes to press, we are preparing to analyze the data from this second pilot study.

Since 1994, we also have become increasingly interested in the influence of ethnicity and of cultural values on caregivers' stress and coping strategies. Chapter 2, written by T. J. McCallum who presently is a doctoral candidate in clinical psychology and aging at USC, summarizes our thinking about ethnic issues, especially with regard to African American caregivers. While still in very early stages of development, we expect that theories of caregiving and interventions to help caregivers (including this one) will need to be adapted to work with different ethnic groups and in other nations.

There are many other people who deserve recognition for contributing to this project. Dozens of graduate and undergraduate students in gerontology, clinical psychology, and social work have worked on the stress reduction project at one time or another since 1989. They drove all over Los Angeles County and sometimes into Orange and Ventura Counties to interview or to teach stress reduction training. And, of course, the caregivers themselves deserve credit for sharing their lives, caregiving experiences, and perceptions of their own stress and coping.

The stress reduction training program for caregivers is still a work in progress. The experience of doing the revised version (the model presented in this volume) generally has seemed positive to us. We have had fewer dropouts and fewer times when we have thought the caregivers have not been applying the techniques in their daily lives, and both trainers and caregivers have seemed more satisfied. Of course, analyzing the data from this second pilot study may lead to more revisions. Before we truly can be confident in recommending the use of this approach, larger scale intervention research is needed.

In the meantime, we offer stress reduction training for caregivers as a developing approach that is strongly grounded in research and theory on caregiving within the stress and coping model and which uses cognitive behavioral techniques that are strongly grounded in research on stress reduction in other populations.

Bob G. Knight

CHAPTER

Stress and Coping Models of Caregiving Distress

Demographic trends in the United States, as in other industrialized countries, show an increase in the relative percentage and absolute numbers of the older population (65+ years old). In 1900, 4% of the population was age 65 or older, whereas by 1990, the percentage had grown to 12.5% (U.S. Bureau of the Census, 1995). In addition, the oldest old segment of the population (85+ years old) will increase dramatically before the year 2000 (National Institute on Aging, 1987). This projection will have several consequences on society, not only in economic terms, but also in the composition of society and in the roles expectation related to the care of older people.

According to Melcher (1988), the increase in life expectancy, the aging of the population, and the advances in medical technology and medicine will lead to an increase in the number of frail older people who will require care from their family or from society. Does the increase in life expectancy imply a higher percentage of disease among the oldest segment of the population? According to Peterson (1994), as a person ages, his or her biological and physiological systems deteriorate. Peterson postulated possible interactions between the aging process and disease; disease is more likely to occur with

This chapter, and especially the introduction to it, was written with the assistance of Elena Fernandez. It draws upon the introduction to her master's thesis in gerontology at USC's Leonard Davis School of Gerontology. Ms. Fernandez is currently a doctoral student in clinical psychology at the Universidad de Barcelona (Catalonia, Spain).

older age. On the other hand, he also supported the premise that aging is not equivalent to disease. Crimmins, Saito, and Ingegneri (1989) has argued that the average period of frailty has remained constant, at about 3 years before death, as life expectancy has increased. Taking as an example the probability of dementia, George, Blazer, Winfield-Laird, Leaf, and Fischbach (1988) estimated the prevalence of mild cognitive impairment at 13% for persons age 65 to 74, increasing to 24% for those age 85 or older.

As the percentage of frail and dependent older people increases, the number of families involved in the care of this segment of the population also increases. Research has found that almost half of older people live with their spouse, while about 15% live with a nonspousal relative (Chappel, 1991). Most help is thought to be provided by unpaid caregivers who are family members and friends. Twenty-nine percent are adult daughters, 23% wives, 12.5% husbands, 8.5% sons, and 27% other relatives (such as siblings or grandchildren) and nonrelatives including sons-in-law or daughters-in-law (Finucane & Burton, 1994).

Family caregivers perform the first line of care for frail older people by providing needed services at home, usually for several years before seeking institutional care (Horowitz, 1985). In the United States, a large number of families take on the responsibility of a family member with a chronic or deteriorating disability or disease. But, what is a family caregiver? Family caregivers can be defined in several ways. Based on the American Association of Retired Persons (AARP) and the Travelers Companies Foundations survey (1988), *caregivers* are defined as individuals who provide unpaid assistance, for at least two instrumental activities of daily living or one activity of daily living within 12 months to a person age 50 or older. This definition is somewhat restrictive, however. Caring for someone includes all types of care—from giving companionship to the patient to providing 24 hours of nursing care. A person may be considered the primary family caregiver because he or she has the *responsibility* to provide or obtain proper care or services for the patient. Such objective definitions do not capture the process by which individuals come to think of themselves as caregivers. We have found that some family members provide a lot of care without having identified themselves as caregivers, whereas others have come to see themselves as highly burdened caregivers while doing little besides worrying about a parent. The system of professional services, self-help groups, and advocacy groups for caregivers undoubtedly plays a role in this labeling process.

In most of the families studied, a primary caregiver has been identified (Lebowitz & Light, 1993). In the White U.S. caregivers who have been the primary focus of research so far, the primary caregiver has been selected according to a hierarchy. If available, the first line of defense is a spouse, then a daughter, and then a daughter-in-law (Gatz, Bengtson, & Blum, 1990; Horowitz, 1985). This selection hierarchy clearly is culturally determined.

In Japan and Korea, the oldest son is responsible for his parents, with the personal care being performed by his wife (Choi, 1993; Sung, 1992). In African American families, spousal caregivers are less common, with care more frequently being provided by children and by extended family or fictive kin (see chapter 2 for more on this point). Aranda and Knight (1997) speculated that, in some other cultures (e.g., U.S. Latinos), it may be more appropriate to think of the family system as the caregiving unit. In other words, the whole notion of primary caregiver rather than shared caregiving responsibility may be culture dependent.

☐ Stress and Coping Models

The simplest model of caregiving distress is to think that caregiving always is stressful, that it is stressful because caregiving is hard work, and that caregiving distress follows a "wear and tear" model. That is, the longer caregiving goes on, the more stressful it becomes. Research has suggested that none of these statements are true. These discoveries have then led to thinking of caregiving in a more complex and more accurate way.

Emotional Distress

In this section, we examine emotional distress outcomes for caregivers and then discuss the less frequently studied links of caregiving stress to perceived physical health and to more objective health measures.

There are estimates that symptoms of emotional distress appear in 85% of caregivers (Rabins, Mace, & Lucas, 1982) and that depressive symptoms appear in over 40% (Cohen et al., 1990; Haley, Levine, Brown, Berry, & Hughes, 1987). Gallagher, Rose, Rivera, and Lovett (1989) used the Schedule for Affective Disorders and Schizophrenia (SADS) interview schedule to diagnose affective disorders in caregivers. Dura, Stukenberg, and Kiecolt-Glaser (1991) used the Diagnostic Interview Schedule (DIS) to diagnose affective and anxiety disorders in caregivers. Caregivers reported higher levels of depression and anxiety than noncaregiver comparison samples. The evidence for higher than normal levels of emotional distress outcomes, including syndromal depression and anxiety seems quite clear, at least for White U.S. caregivers.

However, it is important to note that not all caregivers become emotionally distressed. Most research has been done on caregivers who have been seeking help. Even among help seekers, most caregivers have not reported feeling severely emotionally distressed. When non–help-seeking caregivers have been interviewed, they have shown considerably lower rates of depression and other types of distress. For example, Gallagher et al. (1989) found that about half of help seekers, but only about one in five non–help seekers, were depressed. This selection bias is a common problem in clinical research of all kinds (medical and psychosocial) and simply reflects the reality that people seek help when they are feeling bad. The studies of help-seeking caregivers are valuable in understanding other help-seeking caregivers, but they are not representative of all caregivers, many of whom seem to be doing reasonably well.

Researchers also have found evidence that caregiving can lead to higher levels of life satisfaction (Motenko, 1989). From national estimates in 1987, almost three fourths of all caregivers interviewed reported that the caregiving role made them feel useful, and that it contributed to their self-worth (Schulz, Visintainer, & Williamson, 1990; U.S. House of Representatives, Select Committee on Aging, 1987). To complicate the matter further, some researchers, such as Lawton and his colleagues (Lawton, Moss, Kleban, Glicksman, & Rovine, 1991) reported that caregiving satisfaction and caregiving burden sometimes go hand in hand. That is, caregiving can be both positive and negative at the same time.

Summary

Caregiving appears to operate as a form of chronic stress that makes caregivers more susceptible to emotional distress and to clinical disorders such as depression and anxiety. Caregiving also has a positive dimension, which sometimes is mixed with the emotional distress. One issue, as yet not resolved by research, is whether caregivers develop specific emotional reactions (depression, anxiety, anger) or whether all of these emotions are a part of a more general emotional distress response as occurs with other life stress reactions (Stephens & Hobfoll, 1990). Hooker and her colleagues (Hooker, Monahan, Bowman, Frazier, & Shifren, 1998; Hooker, Monahan, Shifren, & Hutchinson, 1992) have modeled the emotional outcomes of caregiving as a single factor, a result which favors the general distress model and which we have replicated in our research (Fox, Knight, & Chou, 1997). This result would provide theoretical support for psychological interventions that are aimed at stress reactions in general over those aimed at specific emotions.

In our psychoeducational intervention strategies, we attempt to directly reduce the emotional distress reaction by the use of progressive relaxation training (also a key element in Meichenbaum's *Stress Inoculation Training*, 1985) and by increasing relaxing events in the caregiver's life, a strategy adapted from the use of pleasant events in Lewinsohn, Munoz, Youngren, and Zeiss's (1986) intervention for depression. Both of these interventions help to increase positive affect and to decrease negative affect.

Perceived Physical Health

Although less clearly established than emotional distress outcomes, caregivers generally have reported that their perception of their own health is lower than that reported by appropriate matched controls or by population norms for age- and gender-matched groups. Stone, Cafferata, and Sangl (1987) found that caregivers in the Informal Caregivers Survey perceived their health as being worse than did age peers in the U.S. population. Lower perceived health ratings also have been reported by other researchers, including Baumgarten, Battista, Infante-Rivard, Hanley, Becker, and Gauthier (Canada; 1992) and Grafstrom, Fratiglioni, Sandman, and Winblad (Sweden; 1992). Snyder and Keefe (1985) reported that 70% of caregivers in their sample attributed declines in physical health to caregiving. Chenoweth and Spencer (1986) found that 21% of caregivers in their sample reported ill health as a primary reason for institutionalizing a relative with dementia. As discussed by Schulz, O'Brien, Bookwala, and Fleissner (1995), perceived physical health in caregivers seems to be determined by risk factors that are similar to those of the larger population (e.g., lower income, high psychological distress, low social support). The factors specific to caregiving seem to be different than those for emotional distress: cognitive impairment in the recipient rather than behavior problems and a much less clear role for the appraisal of caregiving as burdensome (Schulz et al., 1995).

The connection between perceived physical health and objective health outcomes (such as diseases) is not entirely clear. On the one hand, perceived physical health is clearly related to health status, functional ability, and mortality in longitudinal studies (George, 1996). On the other hand, perceived physical health also is related to depression, the personality factor neuroticism, and to other psychological variables (e.g., Hooker et al., 1992, 1998). The perception of physical health is almost certainly influenced both by actual physical health and by psychological distress.

Objective Health Measures

As noted in two extensive reviews by Schulz and his colleagues (Schulz et al., 1990, 1995), objective reports of caregiver health have been far less clear in showing a health difference. Symptom checklists for physical health, number of diseases, medication use, and medical utilization all have shown tremendous variability across samples, with at least as many nonsignificant differences reported as significant ones. Schulz et al. (1990) noted that the extensive use of convenience samples and the likelihood of selection pressures favoring inclusion of healthy caregivers (both because many caregivers are married and married persons are healthier and because health is a factor in becoming and remaining a caregiver as well as in willingness to participate in research) make the interpretation of this null result inconclusive. At present, the clearest result with regard to objective physical health effects is that aspects of immunological functioning are impaired in caregivers and that this leads to higher levels of respiratory infections (Kiecolt-Glaser, Dura, Speicher, & Trask, 1991; Kiecolt-Glaser et al., 1987).

Summary

In short, caregivers are at higher risk of emotional distress, perceive their health as being impaired, and experience changes in immune functioning and a higher prevalence of infectious diseases. As noted above, not all caregivers experience these problems and some people seem to find caregiving a positive experience. If not all caregivers become distressed, and if some feel good about caregiving, then the obvious question for researchers, professionals, and caregivers is, What makes the difference? In what follows, we explore common ideas about why caregiving would be stressful for at least some caregivers, including that caregiving is hard work and therefore stressful and that certain phases of the course of caregiving are stressful, and return to the stress and coping model with its focus on how caregivers' appraise the experience of caregiving.

☐ Is Caregiving Stressful Because It Is Hard Work?

The simplest way of thinking about the connection between stressors and distress reactions is to expect that distress is worse when the stressors are worse. This does not seem to be the case for caregiving. Total caregiving workload, the care receiver's level of illness or disability, and other objective measures of caregiving stressors are not clearly or strongly related to the caregiver's perception of caregiving as burdensome or to health and mental health outcomes. There are a few exceptions. For White U.S. caregivers, the number of behavior problems in the care receiver usually is related to mental health outcomes, and the level of memory impairment often is related to perceived physical health outcomes (see Schulz et al., 1995). Functional disability, number of hours spent caregiving, duration of illness, number of tasks performed for the care recipient, and other objective measures generally are independent of how the caregiver feels. While there is limited cross-cultural evidence, it appears that these findings may be different for other ethnic groups (see chapter 2).

   As will be seen in the more detailed discussion of stress and coping models below, this finding is not uncommon in psychological research on stress and its outcomes. It is not so much the objective stressors which we face, but our interpretation of them and the resources which we have for dealing with stressors that determine our health and mental health reactions.

☐ The Course of Caregiving Distress

As we suggested above, the most common view is that caregiving should get worse as time goes on. This view is especially compelling when the disease process is chronic and progressive (like most dementing illnesses). However, it is far from clear that this is the case. Haley and Pardo (1989) suggested that caregiving may be most stressful in the middle period of a dementing illness, which is the time with the highest frequency of behavior problems (wandering, suspiciousness, anger, and so forth). Gatz, Bengtson, and Blum (1990) discussed the different potential paths of caregiving distress over time and added another: Caregiving could be like grieving, in which the highest level of distress is at the beginning when the caregiver recognizes the problem and begins to make changes in life to allow for caregiving. Once this adjustment occurs, caregiving could get better over time, because caregivers get better at the job of caregiving. These observations of time courses for caregiving distress, which depart from the wear and tear model, call attention to differing aspects of the caregiving experience that could be experienced as stressful: specific types of problems in caring or adjusting to the diagnosis of the care recipient and to the tasks of caregiving. The focus on what is experienced as stressful about caregiving takes us to the stress and coping model, with its emphasis on the appraisal of experiences as stressful.

☐ Stress and Coping Models and the Intervention Presented in This Volume

The understanding of caregiver distress is based on the stress and coping theory developed by Lazarus and Folkman and their colleagues (Folkman, Lazarus, Pimley, & Novacek, 1987; Lazarus & Folkman, 1984). In general, stress and coping models include the following categories of variables: (a) context variables such as gender, age, socioeconomic status, caregiving history, and relationship of the caregiver to the patient; (b) demands on the caregiver: objective stressors or objective burden; (c) the caregiver's appraisal of demands as stressful or satisfying: subjective caregiver burden; (d) the potential mediators between appraisal and outcomes: coping styles and social support; and (e) the consequences of caregiving demands: emotional distress and health outcomes. (See Figure 1-1.)

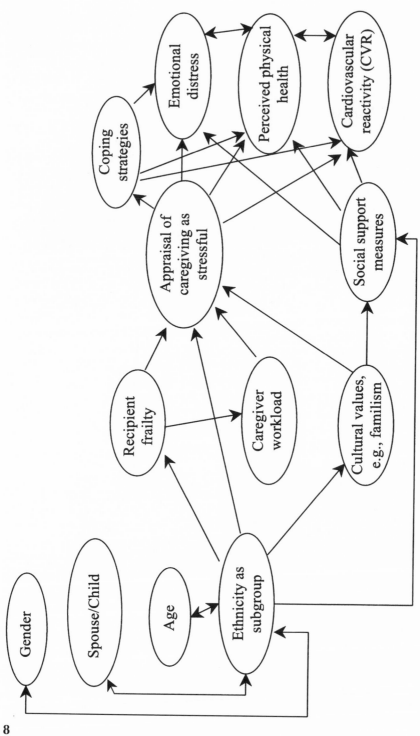

FIGURE 1-1. Sociocultural stress and coping model.

Appraisal of Stressors

A key step in the stress and coping model is appraisal of the situation as stressful or not stressful. Some caregivers obviously appraise (or perceive) caregiving to be highly stressful, whereas others, as discussed above, find it a challenge in a positive sense or even find it enjoyable. Why this is so for different individuals may not always be clear. Cultural values and beliefs likely play a role. Aranda and Knight (1997) argued that the finding that African American caregivers often report lower levels of burden may be due to cultural differences, such as a greater emphasis on family rather than on individuality. In research by Hooker et al. (1998) and in our research, the personality factor neuroticism has been shown to play a role in influencing the appraisal of caregiving as stressful. Individuals high in neuroticism tend to experience negative emotions in response to life stresses, to focus more on their internal reactions, and to often use ineffective coping strategies like avoidance coping (see section below on coping).

Regardless of the reason, this aspect may be changeable, within realistic limits. Ellis (1962; specifically applied to stress reduction in Ellis, Gordon, Neenan, & Palmer, 1997), the originator of a type of cognitive therapy called rational emotive therapy, argued that much emotional distress comes from unrealistically negative appraisals of stressful situations. That is, a person looks at a bad situation and perceives it as a hopeless catastrophe. This also is likely to be true for some caregivers. Many caregiving stressors are undeniably bad (including the fact of a relative with dementia), but caregivers may be able to reduce distress by changing the thoughts that are repeated to themselves about the caregiving and about the illness (see chapter 6).

The relationship of self-talk to stress is also a key component of Stress Inoculation Training as developed by Meichenbaum (1985). Modifying what people say to themselves about objective stressors changes their response to the stress situation. Meichenbaum's approach to cognitive restructuring was more general than that of Ellis, who specifically emphasized the irrationality of thought styles like catastrophizing. In our view, both ways of approaching cognitive restructuring are potential strategies for changing appraisals of caregiving as highly stressful to more neutral.

Coping Styles

Coping styles have long been recognized as an important influence on mental health outcomes among caregivers. Within the stress and coping model, coping styles are mobilized by the appraisal of an objective event as being stressful. Styles of cognitive coping in stressful situations often are more important in determining the emotional response to stress than the objective stressor itself (Folkman et al., 1987; Folkman & Lazarus, 1984; Haley, Levine, Brown, & Bartolucci, 1987). Within the Folkman and Lazarus model, coping styles are generally characterized as active coping (changing or solving the problem situation) or as emotion regulation (changing the emotional reaction to the stressor). Cognitive coping strategies have been strongly related to emotional distress in caregivers of persons with dementia (Haley et al., 1996; Pruchno & Resch, 1989; Stephens, Norris, Kinney, Ritchie, & Grotz, 1988).

While in theory, emotion regulation coping can have positive outcomes, the particular styles studied in caregivers have tended to have negative outcomes, making the emotional distress reaction worse rather than better. Emotion-focused coping styles such as escape-avoidance coping and self-blame have been linked to high levels of emotional distress in caregivers (Fox et al., 1997; Pruchno & Resch, 1989; Stephens et al., 1988). Haley et al. (1996) reported a structural equation model of stress and coping processes in caregivers that showed a significant relationship between avoidance coping and depression. In general, the strategies that are ineffective (e.g., escape-avoidance coping, self-blame) are more clear than the strategies that work, especially for chronic stressors without action-oriented solutions, like caregiving for a family member with dementia.

Very few problems can be solved by avoiding them or wishing they would go away. Accepting responsibility (or, more negatively, self-blame) also is sometimes found to be associated with higher levels of emotional distress in caregivers (Knight, 1992). It seems likely that this coping style may be helpful in some situations (perhaps in working out problems with a cognitively intact spouse or family member), but is not helpful when it amounts to blaming oneself for the problems caused by the dementing illness.

Since avoidance coping does not work, it would be tempting to assume that directly confronting and solving the problems of caregiving would be a good way to avoid emotional distress. However, this coping style often is found to be unrelated to distress outcomes among caregivers. Many of the problems associated with dementia are not really solvable. Vitaliano, De-Wolfe, Maiuro, Russo, and Katon (1990) found that, unlike persons dealing with work problems or physical health problems, dementia caregivers who appraised their stress as changeable reported higher levels of stress. Williamson and Schulz (1993) examined coping among dementia caregivers in a more problem-specific way and reported that some issues respond to problem-solving coping (e.g., seeking social support for coping with the recipient's decline) and others do not (e.g., direct action for problems due to the memory impairment).

We think that the better overall strategy for dementia caregivers is acceptance coping, and some recent data from our research provides preliminary support for this idea. Acceptance coping means accepting a problem rather than avoiding it and then realizing that the situation must be adjusted to rather than actively changed. For the dementia caregiver, this means that the dementia and the changes in the family member will not change. The caregiver can then focus attention on changing his or her reaction to the caregiving stressors rather than trying to solve unsolvable problems. In general, this has been operationalized in our intervention as a guideline for changing self-talk. That is, when altering what caregivers say to themselves about stress events using cognitive restructuring strategies (Ellis et al., 1997; Meichenbaum, 1985), we try to encourage the use of self-statements that reflect acceptance of the reality of the dementia and an acceptance of the behaviors of the person with dementia, as appropriate. Of course, it still is important to solve the specific problems that can be solved.

Social Support

The effects of quantitative social support on caregiver distress are unclear at this time. Caregivers with high levels of support have been found both to be less burdened (Zarit, Reever, & Bach-Peterson, 1980) and more burdened (Knight, 1991; Scott, Roberto, & Hutton, 1986) than other caregivers. Recently, there has been more attention to the costs of social support for caregivers (Schulz, Tompkins, Wood, & Decker, 1987) and to the quality of social support. Conflict with persons in the support system often is linked with high levels of depression (Pagel, Erdly, & Becker, 1987; Rook, 1984).

Many people who should be sources of support are, or are perceived to be, unhelpful and critical of the caregiver. Sometimes there are disagreements about what type of care is needed, how problems should be handled, or even whether the relative has dementia or not. Sometimes advice that is intended to be helpful is taken as criticism because the caregiver already has tried what is being suggested and has found that it does not work.

The relationship between the size of the support network and burden often is positive or zero. It may be that the most important thing is having at least one person who is supportive, and that more is not necessarily better. It may be that quality is more important than quantity. It may be that the relationship works in the opposite direction so that, as caregiving is appraised as being more stressful, the caregiver recruits more helpers into the support network. Highly stressed dementia caregivers may experience stress while maintaining the support system, because persons in the support network expect to receive help and emotional support as well as to provide it, and because support networks also expose members to other people's stress. In any case, it can be useful to keep in mind that not all support is good support, and to maximize the positive and minimize the negative. We only indirectly address changing the social support system, through the focus on monitoring stress and discovering causes of stress (some of which may turn out to be conflicts with presumed social support network members) and increasing the number of relaxing events (which, at least for extroverted caregivers, will involve contact with other people).

☐ Summary

Our intended focus is emotional distress outcomes. As we have discussed earlier in this chapter, it is clear that caregivers have higher levels of emotional distress and higher levels of clinical disorders (like depression and anxiety) than do noncaregivers of similar age and sex. In research from our project (Fox et al., 1997) and in research by Hooker et al. (1992, 1998) emotional distress outcomes for dementia caregivers have been found to be best modeled by a single latent factor of emotional distress. We interpret this as being in support of the view that caregivers, like others responding to severe stressors, experience a wide range of emotional and other responses to that stress. That is, we think it is appropriate to anticipate a variety of emotional distress responses, including depression, anxiety, and hostility, rather than to focus on single emotional responses to caregiving (e.g., on depression only). Thus, in our attempts to help caregivers, we ask them to rate their daily stress level rather than any one emotion, and our targets focus on alleviating stress in general rather than on targeting a specific emotion.

We also mean this to be a specific goal of treatment. That is, our aim is to change emotional outcomes and alleviate the caregiver's felt distress. We do not know if this will affect other outcomes such as health. We believe that interventions specifically aimed at health outcomes will be needed to improve caregiver health, but the research does not support any position on this issue at present.

We also are not convinced that improving the mental health of caregivers necessarily will keep the relative with dementia out of institutional care. A colleague's dissertation research (Lutzky, 1995) found no correlations between stress and coping model variables and decisions to place relatives in institutional care. Clinical experience suggests that sometimes the decision to place the patient is the appropriate decision for all involved. We also have found that reducing emotional distress makes it easier for some caregivers to continue providing care and for others to make the decision that it is time to seek 24-hour care.

In our view, these decisions are highly individual, and most likely are affected by factors other than caregiver emotional distress and the stress and coping model. These observations may explain in part why both psychosocial interventions and respite care seem to help caregivers feel better, but have little or no impact on prolonging family caregiving at home (see Knight, Lutzky & Macofsky-Urban, 1993; Weissert, Cready, & Pawelak, 1988). In any case, our aim is to help caregivers reduce emotional distress, as it is broadly defined. We are not claiming to also do other things.

With these limitations noted, we do feel that the approach described in this volume is helpful in reducing emotional distress when working with caregivers of older adults with dementia. This approach is based on current research knowledge with regard to stress and coping among dementia caregivers. It also draws on long-established psychological intervention techniques from behavioral and cognitive-behavioral approaches to stress reduction. In the chapters that follow, we describe the techniques, the caregivers' individual responses to them, and suggestions for responding to common problems that arise when using these strategies with caregivers.

☐ References

American Association of Retired Persons and Travelers Companies Foundation. (1988). *A national survey of caregivers. Final report. Health advocacy section.* Washington, DC: Opinion Research Corporation.

Aranda, M. P., & Knight, B. G. (1997). The influence of ethnicity and culture on the caregiver stress and coping process: A sociocultural review and analysis. *Gerontologist, 37,* 342–354.

Baumgarten, M., Battista, R. N., Infante-Rivard, C., Hanley, J. A., Becker, R., & Gauthier, S. (1992). The psychological and physical health of family members caring for an elderly person with dementia. *Journal of Clinical Epidemiology, 45,* 61–70.

Chappel, N. (1991). Living arrangements and sources of caregiving. *Journal of Gerontology. Social Sciences, 46,* S1–8.

Chenowith, B., & Spencer, B. (1986). Dementia: The experience of family caregivers. *The Gerontologist, 26,* 267–272.

Choi, H. (1993). Cultural and noncultural factors as determinants of caregiver burden for the impaired elderly in South Korea. *The Gerontologist, 33,* 8–15.

Cohen, D., Luchins, D., Eisdorfer, C., Paveza, G. J., Ashford, J. W., Gorelick, P., Hirschman, R., Freels, S., Levy, P., Semla, T., & Shaw, H. (1990). Caregivng for relatives with Alzheimer's disease: The mental health risks to spouses, adult children and other family members. *Behavior, Health, and Aging, 1,* 171–182.

Crimmins, E., Saito, Y., & Ingegneri, D. (1989). Changes in life expectancy and disability-free life expectancy in the United States. *Population and Development Review, 15,* 235–267.

Dura, J. R., Stukenberg, K. W., & Kiecolt-Glaser, J. (1991). Anxiety and depressive disorders in adult children caring for demented parents. *Psychology and Aging, 6,* 467–473.

Ellis, A. (1962). *Reason and emotion in psychotherapy.* New York: Lyle Stuart.

Ellis, A., Gordon, J., Neenan, M., & Palmer, S. (1997). *Stress counseling: A rational emotive behaviour approach.* London: Cassell.

Finucane, T., & Burton, J. (1994). Community-based long-term care. In W. Hazzard, E. Bierman, J. P. Blass, W. H. Ettinger, Jr., & J. B. Halter (Eds.), *Principles of geriatric medicine and gerontology* (3rd ed.). New Baskerville, USA: McGraw-Hill, Inc.

Folkman, S., Lazarus, R. S., Pimley, S., & Novacek, J. (1987). Age differences in stress and coping processes. *Psychology and Aging, 2,* 171–184.

Fox, L. S., Knight, B. G., & Chou, C. (1997, November). Caregiver burden: Stress appraisal or outcome measure? Presented at the Annual Meeting of the Gerontological Society of America, Cincinnati, OH.

Gallagher, D., Rose, J., Rivera, P., Lovett, S. (1989). Prevalence of depression in family caregivers. *Gerontologist, 29,* 449–456

Gatz, M., Bengston, V. L., & Blum, M. J. (1990). Caregiving families. In J. E. Birren & K. W. Schaie (Eds.), *Handbook of the psychology of aging* (3rd ed.), (pp. 405–426). San Diego, CA: Academic Press.

George, L. (1996). Social factors and illness. In R. Binstock & L. George (Eds.), *Handbook of aging and the social sciences* (4th ed., pp. 229–252). San Diego, CA: Academic Press.

George, L., Blazer, D., Winfield-Laird, I., Leaf, P., & Fischbach, R. (1988). Psychiatric disorders and mental health service use in later life: Evidence from the epidemiological catchment area programs. In J. Brody & G. Maddox (Eds.), *Epidemiology and aging: An international perspective* (pp. 189–219). New York: Springer.

Grafstrom, M., Fratiglioni, L., Sandman. P. O., & Winblad, B. (1992). Health and social consequences for relatives of demented and nondemented elderly: A population-based study. *Journal of Clinical Epidemiology, 45,* 861–870.

Haley, W., Bartolucci, A., Brown, S. L., & Bartolucci, A. A. (1987). Stress, appraisal, coping and social support as predictors of adaptational outcome among dementia caregivers. *Psychology and Aging, 2,* 323–330.

Haley, W. E., Levine, E. G., Brown, S. L., Berry, J. W., & Hughes, G. H. (1987). Psychological, social, and health consequences of caring for a relative with senile dementia. *Journal of the American Geriatrics Society, 35,* 405–411.

Haley, W. E., & Pardo, K. M. (1989). Relationship of severity of dementia to caregiving stressors. *Psychology and Aging, 4,* 389–392.

Haley, W. E., Roth, D. L., Coleton, M. I., Ford, G. R., West, C. A. C., Collins, R. P., & Isobe, T. L. (1996). Appraisal, coping, and social support as mediators of well-being in Black and White family caregivers of patients with Alzheimer's disease. *Journal of Consulting and Clinical Psychology, 64,* 121–129.

Hooker, K., Monahan, D. J., Bowman, S. R., Frazier, L. D., & Shifren, K. (1998). Personality counts for a lot: Predictors of mental and physical health of spouse caregivers in two disease groups. *Journal of Gerontology: Psychological Sciences, 53B,* 75–85.

Hooker, K., Monahan, D., Shifren, K., & Hutchinson, C. (1992). Mental and physical health of caregivers: The role of personality. *Psychology and Aging, 7,* 386–392.

Horowitz, A. (1985). Family caregiving to the frail elderly. *Annual Review of Gerontology and Geriatrics, 5,* 194–246.

Kiecolt-Glaser, J., Dura, J. R., Speicher, C. E., & Trask, O. (1991). Spousal caregivers of dementia victims: Longitudinal changes in immunity and health. *Psychosomatic Medicine, 54,* 345–362.

Kiecolt-Glaser, J., Glaser, R., Shuttleworth, E., Dyer, C., Ogrocki, P., & Speicher, C. (1987). Chronic stress and immunity in family caregivers of Alzheimer's disease victims. *Psychosomatic Medicine, 49,* 523–535.

Knight, B. (1991). Predicting life satisfaction and distress of in-home spouse dementia caregivers. *American Journal of Alzheimer's Care and Research and Related Disorders, 6,* 40–45.

Knight, B. (1992). Emotional distress and diagnosis among helpseekers: A comparison of dementia caregivers and depressed older adults. *Journal of Applied Gerontology, 11,* 361–372.

Knight, B. G., Lutzky, S. M., & Macofsky-Urban, F. (1993). A meta-analytic review of interventions for caregiver distress: Recommendations for future research. *The Gerontologist, 33,* 240–249.

Lawton, M. P., Moss, M., Kleban, M. H., Glicksman, A., & Rovine, M. (1991). A two-factor model of caregiving appraisal and psychological well-being. *Journal of Gerontology, 46,* 181–189.

Lazarus, R. S., & Folkman, S. (1984). *Stress, appraisal, and coping.* New York: Springer.

Lebowitz, B., & Light, E. (1993). Caregiver stress. In T. Yoshikawa, E. L. Cobbs, & K. Brummel-Smith (Eds.), *Ambulatory geriatric care* (pp. 47–54). St. Louis, Mo: Mosby-Year Book, Inc.

Lewinsohn, P., Munoz, R., Youngren, M., & Zeiss, A. (1986). *Control your depression.* Englewood Cliffs, NJ: Prentice Hall.

Lutzky, S. M. (1995). *Understanding of caregiver distress and the decision to place: Applying a stress and coping model.* Unpublished doctoral dissertation, School of Gerontology, University of Southern California, Los Angeles.

Meichenbaum, D. (1985). *Stress inoculation training.* New York: Pergamon Press.

Melcher, J. (1988). Keeping our elderly out of institutions by putting them back in their homes. *American Psychologist, 43,* 643–647.

Motenko, A. (1989). The frustrations, gratifications, and well-being of dementia caregivers. *Gerontologist, 29,* 166–172.

National Institute on Aging (1987). *Personnel for health needs of the elderly through the year 2020.* Bethesda, Maryland: Public Health Services; Department of Health and Human Services.

Pagel, M., Erdly, W., & Becker, J. (1987). Social networks: We get by with (and in spite of) a little help from our friends. *Journal of Personality and Social Psychology, 53,* 793–804.

Peterson, M. (1994). Physical aspects of aging: Is there such a thing as 'normal'?. *Geriatrics, 49,* 45–49.

Pruchno, R. A., & Resch, N. L. (1989). Mental health of caregiving spouses: Coping as mediator, moderator, or main effect? *Psychology and Aging, 4,* 454–463.

Rabins, P., Mace, N. L., & Lucas, M. J. (1982). Impact of dementia on the family. *Journal of the American Medical Association, 248,* 333–335.

Rook, K. S. (1984). The negative side of social interaction: Impact on psychological well-being. *Journal of Personality and Social Psychology, 46,* 1097–1108.

Scott, J. P., Roberto, K. A., & Hutton, T. (1986). Families of Alzheimer's victims: Family support to the caregivers. *Journal of the American Geriatrics Society, 34,* 348–354.

Schulz, R., O'Brien, A. T., Bookwala, J., & Fleissner, K. (1995). Psychiatric and physical morbidity effects of dementia caregiving: Prevalence, correlates, and causes. *Gerontologist, 35,* 771–791.

Schulz, R., Tompkins, C. A., Wood, D., & Decker, S. (1987). The social psychology of caregiving: Physical and psychological costs of providing support to the disabled. *Journal of Applied Social Psychology, 17,* 401–428.

Schulz, R., Visintainer, P., & Williamson, G. M. (1990). Psychiatric and physical morbidity effects of caregiving. *Journal of Gerontology, 45,* 181–191.

Snyder, B., & Keefe, K. (1985). The unmet needs of family caregivers for frail and disabled adults. *Social Work in Health Care, 19,* 1–13.

Stephens, M. A. P., & Hobfoll, S. E. (1990). Ecological perspectives on stress and coping in later-life families. In M. A. P. Stephens, J. H. Crowther, S. E. Hobfoll, & D. L. Tennenbaum (Eds.), *Stress and coping in later-life families* (pp. 287–304). New York: Hemisphere.

Stephens, M. A. P., Norris, V. K., Kinney, J. M., Ritchie, S. W., & Grotz, R. C. (1988). Stressful situations in caregiving: Relations between caregiver coping and well-being. *Psychology and Aging, 3,* 208–209.

Stone, R., Cafferata, G. L., & Sangl, J. (1987). Caregivers of the frail elderly: A national profile. *The Gerontologist, 27,* 616–626.

Sung, K. (1992). Motivations for parent care: The case of filial children in Korea. *International Journal of Aging and Human Development, 34,* 109–124.

U.S. Bureau of the Census. (1995). *Sixty-five plus in the United States.* Washington, DC: U.S. Government Printing Office.

Vitaliano, P. P., DeWolfe, D. J., Maiuro, R. D., Russo, J., & Katon, W. (1990). Appraised changeability of a stressor as a modifier of the relationship between coping and depression: A test of the hypothesis of fit. *Journal of Personality and Social Psychology, 59,* 582–592.

Weissert, W. G., Cready, C. M., & Pawelak, J. (1988). The past and future of home and community based long term care. *The Milbank Quarterly, 66,* 309–388.

Williamson, G. M., & Schulz, R. (1993). Coping with specific stressors in Alzheimer's disease caregiving. *Gerontologist, 6,* 747–755.

Zarit, S. H., Reever, K., & Bach-Peterson, J. (1980). Relatives of the impaired elderly: Correlates of feelings of burden. *Gerontologist, 20,* 373–377.

2

CHAPTER   T. J. McCallum

Dementia Caregiver Burden and Ethnicity

While the literature on caregiving in general continues to expand, research on caregiving among ethnic minorities remains notably limited. When differentiated by specific ethnicity, this lack becomes even more apparent. Within the past several years, only a handful of studies investigating Latino and Asian caregivers in the United States have been published. Studies on African American caregivers, still few and far between, total more than that of any other ethnic group. It is due to this dearth of research on varied minorities that this chapter is limited to a discussion of African American caregivers. Accordingly, although the chapter admittedly is incomplete, it represents an analysis of the most comprehensive body of existing literature on minority caregivers.

For nearly 20 years, caring for an older relative with dementia has been recognized as a source of burden for the caregiver (Zarit, Reever, & Bach-Peterson, 1980). In addition, as the caregiving career can span decades, the process has become a prime exemplar of the effects of chronic stress on physical health and mental health outcomes. The literature documenting the effects of caregiving on self-report emotional distress largely has been a literature of White caregivers in the United States (Schulz, O'Brien, Bookwalla, & Fleissner, 1995). Results from a number of research studies, on the other hand, strongly suggest that African American caregivers appraise caregiving as less burdensome than do White caregivers (Fredman, Daly, & Lazur, 1995; Lawton, Rajagopal, Brody, & Kleban, 1992; Morycz, Malloy,

Bozich, & Martz 1987). At present, few researchers have investigated the social, psychological, and physiological aspects associated with dementia caregiving in general, and particularly in the African American community. Accompanying this research void is a lack of theoretical models to account for these differences (Dilworth-Anderson & Anderson, 1994), with the exception of recent studies by Haley et al. (1995, 1996) and Knight and McCallum (1998).

According to Dilworth-Anderson and Anderson (1994), any model attempting to investigate caregiver stress in the African American population should examine sociocultural factors such as social supports and strains, psychological factors such as coping resources, and physiological change factors such as cardiovascular reactivity (CVR). This chapter is an attempt to bring together the present research connecting these factors in relation to the African American caregiver and stress.

☐ Sociocultural Factors and Social Support

There are a wide variety of sociocultural factors that differentiate African Americans and Whites in this country, such as years of education, employment, and geographical distribution. In the realm of caregiving, however, several similarities among ethnicities should be noted. Most caregivers are women, many are not married and are of low income, and many report being in fair to poor health (Fredman et al., 1995; Haley, Levine, Brown, & Bartolucci, 1987; Knight & McCallum, 1998).

Some have argued that social support is a conceptual offshoot of extended families and is fundamental to well-being in the African American community (Neighbors, 1997). *Social support,* defined here as those interpersonal transactions involving aid, affect, or affirmation (Kahn & Antonucci, 1980), has been extensively examined in the context of caregiving over the past two decades. Within this context, a number of studies investigating the social support networks of African American caregivers, as well as a few on network comparisons between African American and White caregivers have been conducted. Despite evidence of more variation within social support networks (Burton et al., 1995; Gibson, 1982), African American caregiver networks have not been shown to be significantly larger than those of White caregivers (Burton et al., 1995; Haley et al., 1995). This chapter examines the factors most relevant to caregiving according to Dilworth-Anderson and Anderson (1994): the cultural characteristics (cultural tradition, family dynamics, the role of the church) and coping style of African Americans.

☐ Cultural Tradition

Many cultural characteristics of African Americans can be traced to African culture and traditions (Nobles, 1980). One such African tradition present in African American culture is the importance of the extended family, which often includes both blood relatives and non–blood-related individuals who may be given similar status to blood relatives (Nobles, 1974). This is in sharp contrast to the concept of the nuclear family prevalent in White American culture, a concept which may create clear and distinct roles for relatives and lesser or nonexistent roles for those outside of the immediate family. These group differences in familial organization may begin to explain differences in caregiving.

Lawton et al. (1992) examined "traditional caregiving ideology," and found that African Americans scored higher than Whites in this category (although it should be noted that traditional caregiving ideology did not correlate with burden). Traditional caregiving ideology is based on the Barresi and Menon (1990) notion that African Americans are socialized or inculcated with attitudes that encourage providing respect and assistance to older family members. Lawton et al. (1992) described the ideology as continuing a family tradition of mutual concern.

This suggestion of a stronger mutual concern within the African American community has been described by Johnson and Barer (1990). In their study of older inner-city African Americans and Whites selected from medical clinics, they found that the former group had a more active social support network. The authors employed focused interview techniques involving open-ended questions which, due to questionable validity, are more common to theoretical rather than empirical research, and did not report validity coefficients. Their measures regarding support networks lacked necessary detail, particularly in the area of emotional support. Information about overall mood also was extracted from life review techniques. This information suggested that mechanisms within African American families which serve to expand network membership in two distinct ways. Networks expand through the mobilization of relatives on the periphery of the kinship network (cousins, nieces, and nephews), and through the extension of the kinship network through the creation of *fictive kin*, or individuals given the status and responsibilities of relatives who are not blood relations. A 1995 study found that older disabled African Americans had a greater likelihood of having at least one caregiver who was not part of the immediate family, controlling for variables such as network size (Burton et al., 1995). While Burton et al. found no differences in the total size of social support network, there were significant differences between the two populations that call into question their comparability and thus the generalizability of these results.

African Americans in this study were younger, had significantly less education, and over half lived under the poverty line. Also, reported cognitive status differences were vast, with 46% of the African Americans scoring in the impaired range of the brief screening instrument versus only 25% of the Whites. Though the authors noted the potential confound with level of education on their cognitive function measure, the Short Portable Mental Status Questionnaire, a more comprehensive measure of cognitive function should have been employed. Despite these differences and limitations, this study does support the idea of a more varied network of support among older African Americans based on the aforementioned methods of expansion. For example, grandparents may raise the offspring of distant relatives or friends who, in later life, may come to serve as caregivers even though they do not possess biological ties. Such fictive kin may serve important emotional and instrumental needs for older African Americans that biological relations may not. While fictive kin may have its roots in African tradition, its present day use also can be connected to the relationship dynamics in African American families.

☐ Family Dynamics

Over the past few decades, major trends affecting African American family structure, such as increases in cohabitation and nonmarital births, delays in marriage formation, marriage dissolution, and remarriage and an increase in the number of blended families in this country have impacted and altered family dynamics in African American families. Longitudinal studies examining the African American family have found that Blacks are more likely than Whites to live in extended family households. Furthermore, there is some evidence that one of the benefits of the extended family is the ability to care for impaired family members (Taylor, Tucker, Chatters, & Jayakody, 1997). Factors such as the increase in the number of births to unmarried women, the subsequent rise in the number of female-headed families, the increase in coresident living arrangements in female-headed families, and the rise in never-married African Americans. Other factors include increased cohabitation and the increase in multigenerational households not directly defined by blood linkages. Generally, cohabiting unions are less stable and of shorter duration than legal marriages (Bumpass, Sweet, & Cherlin, 1991), furthermore, African American cohabitating couples are a great deal more likely than White cohabitating couples to have children (McLanahan & Casper, 1995). According to Johnson and Barer (1990), the results of their study of families and networks among older, inner-city African Americans reflect the lack of stable, long-term marriages in the inner-city African American community, with only 14% of their sample reporting currently being married or cohabiting. Over half of their sample reported being divorced, and many within that group reported multiple marriages. High divorce rates and multiple marriages create a network of relatives that may become quite flexible and able to adapt to the needs of those within the system. In the context of caregiving, this results in fewer spouse and blood-related caregivers than in the White caregiving population. The 1992 Lawton et al. study reported that far fewer African American caregivers (27.3%) were spouses, as compared with the White sample (51.2%), and that many more African American caregivers either were other relatives (not children-in-law or siblings) or friends (17.6% vs. 4.2%). Haley et al. (1995) found similar distributions of spouses and adult children in the caregiving role, and also reported that the percentage of divorced caregivers in their study was eight times higher for African American caregivers (25%) than for White caregivers (3%). For older African Americans, this extended family network system provides a greater number of relatives from which to choose when assistance is needed, and this may partially explain the large number of nonspousal, nonchild caregivers within the African American community. The following case example outlines the life of one such African American nonspousal, grandchild caregiver.

☐ Case Example

Ms. Carson

Ms. Carson is a single African American woman in her late thirties who serves as a caregiver for her 76-year-old grandmother. Ms. Carson's caregiving role began 3 years ago, after her aunt suffered a fatal stroke. Her aunt had lived with her grandmother for 20 years, the past 4 as a caregiver. Ms. Carson's grandmother was diagnosed with probable Alzheimer's disease 7 years ago.

Ms. Carson previously had been a secondary caregiver, assisting her aunt in the care of her grandmother on weekends and after work. Though she lived about 40 miles from her older relatives, Ms. Carson considered it to be her familial duty to help out as much as possible. She decided to move in with her grandmother after her aunt's death, despite the fact that the once nice neighborhood had deteriorated badly. Her grandmother's large old house also was in need of many repairs.

Ms. Carson had worked full time for a large metropolitan newspaper for 15 years, and finally had to take an unpaid leave of absence to stay with her grandmother. Over the past 3 years, she had used up all of her vacation and sick leave to assist her grandmother with various appointments and to repair parts of the house.

As the only grandchild in contact with her deceased mother's side of the family, Ms. Carson believes it is her duty to care for her grandmother. She feels strongly about caring for her grandmother herself, despite suggestions from several of her friends that she place her grandmother in a nursing home.

The behavior of her grandmother is erratic, but Ms. Carson handles it quite well. The pair maintain a very regimented schedule, which seems to help reduce the grandmother's general confusion. The biggest problems faced by Ms. Carson include her grandmother's unpredictable angry and violent tirades, her grandmother's attempt to cook despite having started two fires by leaving food on the stove and forgetting about it, and her grandmother's sleeplessness. Ms. Carson has the most difficulty in encouraging her grandmother to sleep through the night, and reports that her own sleeplessness is beginning to wear her down physically.

Ms. Carson's social life has suffered somewhat over the past 3 years, but she did not engage in a large number of social events before her life as a primary caregiver. Her long-time boyfriend understands and has accepted the change. Although the couple's dates are less frequent now, they speak on the phone every day, which is more often than they had done previously.

The church has become central in the lives of both Ms. Carson and her grandmother. Not only do they attend church together on Sundays, but many members of the church assist Ms. Carson in various ways. Members visit several times a week to allow Ms. Carson time for grocery shopping and an occasional movie, and other caregivers from the church have created a phone network to check up on each other a few times a week.

Ms. Carson's grandmother remains in excellent physical health, and may live for another 20 years. Through her religious faith, Ms. Carson accepts her role and the difficulties inherent in it. She does not intend to place her grandmother in a nursing home, unless her grandmother requires medical assistance that she cannot provide. Though small, her social support system, fulfills her needs at the present time.

☐ The Role of the Church

An additional source of assistance for older African Americans is the church, the importance of which reflects another cultural remnant from Africa that has ramifications for caregiving. The church, along with support from family and friends, composes a mutual aid system for many older African Americans. Within the mutual aid system, older African Americans and their adult children provide care and support to each other, at higher rates than do older Whites and their offspring (Mutran, 1985). Walls and Zarit (1991) also concluded that African American churches serve as a strong support network for older African Americans. Although they found that the family was the strongest source of support, the informal networks derived through the church tended to complement that support, with both networks predicting well-being. The church, therefore, may add both qualitative and quantitative social support to older African Americans. Last, there is evidence that the church also facilitates the utilization of specific coping styles in the African American community.

☐ Caregiver Ethnicity and Coping Style

Just as social support is hypothesized to differentiate African American and White caregivers, there is some evidence that coping style also may differentiate the groups. Past research in the field has demonstrated that a caregiver's negative appraisal of the situation, more than specific situational characteristics, leads to distress and depression (Picot, Debanne, Namazi, & Wykle, 1997). It follows that the style or method by which caregivers cope may be linked to their appraisal of the situation and, in the case of caregiving, perhaps to their view of illness.

According to Landrine and Klonoff (1992), important cultural differences in health-related beliefs and schemas exist between African Americans and Whites, in that many Whites tend to view illness as a person-centered, temporally bounded, and discontinuous event, whereas many ethnic and cultural minority groups in the United States view illness as a long-term, fluid, and continuous manifestation of changing relationships and dysfunctions in the family, the community, or nature. Landrine and Klonoff further suggested that many minority groups view treatment as a long-term, informal, highly personal, and cooperative process in which the healer, victim, and family atone for the wrongdoing and improve the habits and relationships that are construed to be the cause of illness. This view may begin to explain differences between African American and White caregivers in the perception and appraisal of stress in the caregiving role. In other words, if African Americans view dementing illness as fluid and long term, and Whites view the illness as discrete, then African American caregivers may adjust better psychologically to the role strains inherent in long-term caregiving.

A number of caregiving researchers have found several differences between African American and White caregivers which support the idea that African American caregivers do in fact appraise the caregiving role differently than do White caregivers. Morycz, Malloy, Bozich, and Martz (1987) found that African American caregivers experienced less strain, were less likely to institutionalize, and differed from White caregivers in the factors that predicted burden. Fredman et al. (1995) reported similar findings in relation to burden, despite the fact that the African American caregivers in their study reported caring for people with greater functional and cognitive impairment. In their 1992 study, Lawton et al. found that African American caregivers scored higher than White caregivers on scales of mastery and satisfaction, and scored lower on scales designed to test subjective burden, sense of intrusion, and depression. Most recently, Haley and his colleagues (1995) found a higher incidence of depression and decreased life satisfaction in White caregivers when compared with African American caregivers. Knight and McCallum (1998) also found similar evidence of differences in the appraisal of caregiving between ethnicities.

However, according to Lazarus and Folkman (1984), appraisal of a situation is only part of the equation when facing a stressor. Individuals also actively choose how to cope when placed in a potentially stressful situation. The coping style literature contains precious little research on older African Americans, and even less on ethnic caregiving. Nevertheless, work which has been done suggests that older African Americans employ coping styles quite different from older Whites. Picot et al. (1997) found significant differences in the relationship between caregiver ethnicity and the perceived rewards and comfort attained from prayer. This is not surprising in light of earlier findings from religiosity studies indicating higher levels of religiosity among African Americans, females, and older adults (Chatters, Levin, & Taylor, 1992). Specifically, the group found that African American caregivers scored higher on prayer and comfort from religion scales. This result lead Picot et al. (1997) to suggest that religiosity serves as a coping resource variable, which in turn operates as a stress deterrent, as opposed to a stress buffer (Wheaton, 1985). As a resource variable, the function of religious coping may be to raise the African American caregiver's threshold for stress. African American caregivers in this study prayed more frequently, a behavior which may have preceded their caregiving career, and therefore they may have perceived less stress than White caregivers when confronted by the same caregiving situation. Similarly, Krause and Van Tran (1992) found that older African Americans use religious involvement as a counterbalance to offset deleterious effects of stressful circumstances. Though their research indicated that life stresses tended to erode feelings of mastery and self-worth, the negative effects were offset when religious involvement was high. In a study of older African Americans, Neighbors and his colleagues found prayer to be the most frequently mentioned coping resource utilized among this group when faced with a serious personal problem. They also found that the tendency to report prayer as most helpful was highest among those with the most severe personal problems and that, after physicians, ministers were ranked highest among professionals from whom to seek help. Although the aforementioned study did not examine it directly, one need not jump far to make the connection to coping with caregiving as a serious personal problem.

Religious coping also has been considered a path through which African American caregivers cognitively redefine a stressful situation (Skaff, 1995). *Cognitive redefinition*, also known as positive reappraisal, is the act of reframing a potentially stressful event into a more positive light. Though theorized to be utilized more frequently by African Americans, little empirical work has been done on the subject. In perhaps the only study to examine this type of coping with African American caregivers, Knight and McCallum (1998), found significant differences between African American and White caregivers. African American caregivers were found to use positive reappraisal more often than their White counterparts. Furthermore, they found evidence that this coping style may not be useful for Whites. In the study, caregivers of both ethnicities that showed significant CVR levels during two stressful tasks were compared. As expected, positive reappraisal and depression were inversely related for African Americans when the subject shared a stressful story about caregiving. Surprisingly, White caregivers showed a positive relationship between positive reappraisal and depression in both stress conditions. In other words, positive reappraisal appeared to be an effective coping style for African American caregivers, but positively correlated with depression for White caregivers.

The evidence that African American caregivers appraise and cope with the stress inherent in the caregiving role differently than White caregivers is mounting. Positive reappraisal and religious coping are two related styles of coping with the stresses of caregiving that may be used more often and with greater success by African American caregivers than by their White counterparts. Furthermore, the connection between positive reappraisal, CVR, and caregiver ethnicity is important for two reasons. First, it connects physiological measures with psychological ones, adding information not obtainable through paper-and-pencil measures, which in turn adds incremental validity to caregiving research as a whole. Second, the finding that African American caregivers show an inverse relationship to CVR when using positive reappraisal, while White caregivers show a positive relationship between the two, indicates that this particular style of coping may be more useful to reduce stress in one group than the other. In other words, White caregivers may not be able to successfully apply the techniques that seem to aid African American caregivers in reducing caregiving stress. It follows that researchers now entertain the possibility that efficacious stress reduction techniques may differ between these two groups.

☐ Theoretical Explanations

There have been a number of theoretical explanations put forth to explain the paradox of lower reported burden in African American caregivers.

Dilworth-Anderson and Anderson (1994) suggested that caregiving may not be the most salient stressor for many low-income African Americans. Financial stress, child rearing, or job stress may be more important than caregiving in some instances. In attempting to explore these issues, Haley et al. (1996) recently examined stress appraisal, coping, and social support as mediators of well-being in African American and White caregivers. They concluded that the stress process was similar in African American and White caregivers, but suggested that "cultural mechanisms" may explain why the former group appraised and coped with stress more effectively than the latter group. Thus, some aspect of African American culture may facilitate the more effective use of social support or the development of a coping style that differs from White caregivers allowing for more effective coping and, consequently, less burden. Dilworth-Anderson and Anderson (1994) suggested that aspects of caregiving also may increase a personal sense of mastery or increase family cohesiveness in light of a lifetime of other stressors, thus shedding more light on cultural mechanisms at work. The Haley et al. (1996) study found no significant differences in social support, however. Without an empirical link to social support in ethnic caregiving research, the literature simply is unable to explain these consistent ethnic differences in caregiver burden.

Knight and McCallum (1998) hypothesized that reporting bias may explain the ethnic differences in caregiver burden. These authors sought to examine physiological measures of stress in order to compare the two ethnicities and determine if comparable physiological stress measures would indicate that African Americans actually were experiencing similar stress from a physiological vantage point, but were reporting lower levels of stress on psychological inventories. The results of this study did not support such a conclusion. However, more studies attempting to connect physiological stress with psychological stress may uncover some, thus far, elusive answers.

☐ Stress Buffering

Stress researchers have long noted that some individuals are more psychologically vulnerable or responsive to stress than others, even if exposed to similar types or levels of stressors. Further research has suggested that people connected with strong family and friendship networks are less susceptible to the effects of stress and, therefore, are more likely to enjoy higher levels of mental health (Cohen & Willis, 1985). Networks of friends and families are hypothesized to protect members by providing them with emotional or tangible resources that are used to cope with problems or difficulties. While research in the African American community has shown the existence of and importance of elaborate social networks, including extended family, friends, and church members (Chatters, Taylor, & Jackson, 1986), only scant evidence exists in support of a buffering effect against stress.

☐ Physiological Research

As mentioned above, researchers have been examining the effects of caregiving for the past 20 years. When compared to age-matched peers, predominantly White samples of caregivers consistently have been shown to exhibit more depressive symptoms, higher rates of burden, and more perceived hassles (Haley et al., 1987). Lacking in the literature, thus far, have been objective examinations of the physical toll exacted by caregiving as measured by specific physiological markers. Recent studies of immune response and metabolic changes are two avenues by which the physiological effects of caregiving are just beginning to be investigated. This underdeveloped area of research is important not only in that it adds to the cannon of general caregiving literature, but also because it may help shed further light on the consistent and inadequately explained finding of ethnic differences in caregiver burden.

☐ Caregiving and Physiological Stress: A Review of the Literature

Studies of caregiving historically have focused on a variety of concepts of stress. Dozens of models and measures which were designed to explain the impact of stress on the caregiver presently are in use. Researchers, while citing the importance of both mental and physical aspects of stress, often employ measures insufficient to the task of investigating the physiological components of stress, particularly when comparing health outcomes. This is a criticism relevant to the majority of caregiving studies cited in the earlier sections of this chapter. The following is a review of several recent studies that attempt to connect caregiver stress with immunity and metabolic function.

Kiecolt-Glaser, Esterling, and their colleagues have been at the forefront of examining specific health outcomes of caregiving. In a 1987 study, Kiecolt-Glaser et al. conducted one of the first experiments linking caregivers and chronic physiological stress. Theorizing that the long-term stressor of caregiving may have an adverse impact on the immune system, Kiecolt-Glaser et al. compared a predominantly White sample of Alzheimer's caregivers with matched controls employing immunological analyses. They found that caregivers had significantly lower percentages of T lymphocytes and helper T lymphocytes, as well as significantly lower helper suppressor cell ratios. The results suggest that caregivers or, more specifically, White caregivers, possess poorer immunologic adaptation than noncaregivers. Of course, only studies including African American caregivers would validate this finding for that group.

In 1991, Kiecolt-Glaser, Dura, Speicher, Trask, and Glaser launched a longitudinal study in order to examine caregiver immunity and health over time. Again, it is assumed that this study included a predominantly White sample as most of the literature in this realm does not note ethnicity. Between the initial intake and the approximate 13 months later, caregivers showed decrements in immunity and more infectious illness, particularly upper respiratory infection. The study also found that caregivers who reported lower levels of social support at intake and who were most distressed by dementia-related behaviors showed significantly negative changes in immune function at follow up. The connection of social support indicators with aspects of immune function is noteworthy, as this is the first example of an essentially psychosocial indicator having been shown to correspond with a purely physiological measure.

Three years later (Esterling, Kiecolt-Glaser, Bodnar, & Glaser, 1994), the group expanded their scope to examine former and present caregivers, as well as controls along the dimensions of stress and social support. Here they sought to determine whether or not problems such as anxiety, depression, and slowed-down immune system regulation would subside for caregivers with the death of the patient. They found that former caregivers were immunologically indistinguishable from present caregivers. Both groups were significantly more depressed and displayed a poorer immune system response than the controls.

The findings of the previous study were replicated a year later. Castle, Wilkins, Heck, Tanzy, and Fahey (1995) also examined caregivers and immunity. They likewise concluded that a link exists between chronic stress and a lowered immune response which, when adding the variable of age, may combine to increase the risk of disease for caregivers. However, similar to their psychologically and sociologically oriented brethren, these researchers failed to include strong measures from the other realms, rendering their results difficult to generally apply.

Similarly, Mills et al. (1997) matched caregivers and controls while looking at plasma catecholine levels and lymphocyte receptor alterations. They found the chronic stress of caregiving to relate to changes in receptor physiology, and suggested that such stress may alter cellular immunity.

Using all White samples, other researchers also have reported immunological differences between caregivers and noncaregivers. Recently, Vitaliano, Russo, Young, Teri, and Maiuro (1996) investigated the links between metabolic variables, stress, and caregiving. Employing a longitudinal design and a chronic stress perspective, these researchers measured insulin and glucose in caregivers and noncaregiving controls twice over a 15- to 18-month period. They found that caregivers had significantly higher insulin levels than controls at intake and time 2, even when variables of obesity, gender, exercise, age, alcoholic drinks, hormone replacement therapy, lipids, and hypertension were considered in the analysis. They also found psychological distress to be positively associated with glucose at time 2. While Vitaliano et al. did include controls and incorporated strong psychological measures, they did not include any African American caregivers in their study.

In contrast, Knight and McCallum (1998), recently conducted a study investigating ethnic differences in burden, which incorporated commonly used measures from sociological, psychological, and physiological realms. The main findings, mentioned above, suggested that positive reappraisal may be an effective coping style for African American caregivers, but not for Whites. The relationship to positive reappraisal was unexpectedly positive for Whites, with higher reported use of positive reappraisal leading to higher levels of CVR and corresponding with high levels of depression, rather than providing the protective effect as in African Americans. For African American caregivers, the inverse relationship was found.

☐ Caregiving and Poor Health Outcomes

Evidence for the negative impact of physiological caregiving stress on health outcomes is mounting, though it is based on predominantly White caregiving samples. While some may argue that the process of aging alone leads to some of the immunity and metabolic changes suggested by the aforementioned studies, it cannot explain significant differences found between the age-matched controls and the caregivers. In other words, these studies strongly suggested that, due to the stress of caregiving, caregivers may enter higher health risk categories than those dictated by age alone. Specifically, this cross section of studies suggests that caregivers possess poorer immunologic adaptation than noncaregivers, that caregivers show more infectious illness than noncaregivers, and that former caregivers are immunologically indistinguishable from present caregivers.

At present, the physiological caregiving research remains in its infancy as it just begins to empirically examine physiological forms of stress related to caregiving. In some sense, this is where the field of research began 20 years ago. There are, however, some important differences. The caregiving research incorporating physiological information today can benefit from and add to the existing sociological and psychological findings of the past 20 years. In doing so, physiological research holds the key to many advancements in the study of caregiver burden and can elucidate information that exists on ethnic differences.

☐ Summary

Historically, little research has been conducted investigating African American caregivers and stress. The research which has been done can be divided into three distinct areas: sociological research, psychological research, and, more recently, physiological research. In the sociological realm, the social support research conducted has underlined the importance of cultural traditions of an expanded kinship network, the complex family dynamics marked by divorce and multigenerational households, and the role of the church in facilitating and supplementing this family system in relation to caregiving. Researchers in psychology have explored differences in the view of illness and in coping style between African American caregivers and their White counterparts, concluding that both factors impact the stress appraisal process in a manner that may begin to explain why African American caregivers report lower burden in the caregiving role. The physiological research has included few African American participants, but suggests that caregivers are at greater health risks due to poorer immune function. Perhaps the most consequential work that has been done thus far, however, combines aspects of these three areas. Kiecolt-Glaser et al.'s (1991) work connecting poor immune function to low social support and the Knight and McCallum (1998) study linking coping style to CVR serve as examplars of the next step in this line of research.

The ultimate benefit of this line of research would be seen in the creation of models of caregiver stress that would isolate the points of impact wherein stress reduction techniques can be employed. Simultaneously, researchers can work to determine if physiological system function parallels that of the complex emotional system that leads to caregiver burden. In other words, they can explore the possibility that social support and coping style directly impact immune function. As consistent reporters of low levels of burden, continued integrated research on African American caregivers and stress is paramount if these goals are to be realized.

☐ References

Barresi, C., & Menon, G. (1990). Diversity in Black family caregiving. In Z. Harel, E. Mc Kinney, & M. Williams (Eds.), Black Aged (pp. 221–235). Newbury Park, CA: Sage.

Bumpass, L., Sweet, J., & Cherlin, A. (1991). The role of cohabitation in declining rates of marriage. *Journal of Marriage and the Family, 53*, 913–927.

Burton, L., Kasper, J., Shore, A., Cagney, K., La Veist, T., Cubbin, C., & German, P. (1995). The structure of informal care: Are there differences by race? *The Gerontologist, 35*, 744–752.

Castle, S., Wilkins, S., Heck, E., Tanzy, K., & Fahey, J. (1995). Depression in caregivers of demented patients is associated with altered immunity: Impaired proliferative capacity, increased CD8, and a decline in lymphocytes with surface signal transduction molecules and a cytotoxicity marker. *Clinical Experimental Immunology, 101*, 487–493.

Chatters, L., Taylor, R, & Jayakody, R. (1994). Fictive kin relationships in Black extended families. *Journal of Comparative Family Studies, 25*, 297–312.

Chatters, L., Levin, J., & Taylor, R. (1992). Antecedents and dimensions of religious involvement among older Black adults. *Journal of Gerontology: Social Sciences, 47*, S269–S278.

Chatters, L., Taylor, R., & Jackson, R. (1986). Aged black's choice for an informal helper network. *Journal of Gerontology, 41*, 94–100.

Cohen, S., & Wills, T. (1985). Stress, social support, and the buffering process. *Psychological Bulletin, 98*, 310–357.

Dilworth-Anderson, P., & Anderson, N. B. (1994). Dementia caregiving in Blacks: A contextual approach to research. In B. Lebowitz, E. Light, & G. Niederehe (Eds.), Stress effects on family caregivers of Alzheimer's patients (pp. 385–409). New York: Springer.

Esterling, B., Kiecolt-Glaser, J., Bodnar, J., & Glaser, R. (1994). Chronic stress, social support persistent alterations in the natural killer cells response to cytokines in older adults. *Health Psychology, 13 (4)*, 291–298.

Fredman, L., Daly, M., & Lazur, A. (1995). Burden among White and Black caregivers to elderly adults. *Journals of Gerontology: Social Sciences, 50*, 110–118.

Gibson, R. (1982). Blacks at middle and late life: Resources and coping. *Annals of the American Academy of Political and Social Science, 464*, 79–90.

Haley, W., Levine, E., Brown, S., & Bartolucci, A. (1987). Stress, appraisal, coping, and social support as predictors of adaptational outcome among dementia caregivers. *Psychology and Aging, 2*, 323–330.

Haley, W., Roth, D., Coleton, M., Ford, G., West, C., Collins, R., & Isobe, T. (1996). Appraisal, coping, and social support as mediators of well being in Black and White family caregivers of patients with Alzheimer's disease. *Journal of Consulting and Clinical Psychology, 64*, 121–129.

Haley, W., West, C., Wadley, V., Ford, G., White, Barrett, J., Harrell, L., & Roth, D. (1995). Psychological, social, and health impact of caregiving: A comparison of Black and White dementia family caregivers and noncaregivers. *Psychology and Aging, 10*, 540–552.

Jackson, J., Jayakody, R., & Antonucci, T. (1996). Exchanges within Black American three generation families: The family environment context model. *Journal of Marriage and the Family, 55*, 261–276.

Johnson, C., & Barer, B. (1990). Families and networks among older inner-city Blacks. *The Gerontologist, 30*, 726–733.

Kahn, R., & Antonucci, T. (1980). Convoys over the life course: Attachment, roles, and social support. In P. Baltes and O. Brim (Eds.), Life-span development and behavior (Vol. 3, pp. 253–286). Lexington, MA: Lexington Books.

Kiecolt-Glaser, J., Dura, J., Speicher, C., Trask, O., & Glaser, R. (1991). Spousal caregivers of dementia victims: Longitudinal changes in immunity and health. *Psychosomatic Medicine, 53*, 345–362.

Kiecolt-Glaser, J., Glaser, R., Shuttleworth, E., Dyer, C., Ogrocki, P., & Speicher, C. (1987). Chronic stress and immunity in family caregivers of Alzheimer's disease patients. *Psychosomatic Medicine, 49*, 523–535.

Knight, B., & McCallum, T. (1998). Heart rate reactivity and depression in African-American and White dementia caregivers: Reporting bias or positive coping? *Aging and Mental Health, 2*, 212–221.

Krause, N. (1992). Stress, religiosity, and psychological well-being among older Blacks. *Journal of Aging and Health, 4*, 412–439.

Landrine, H., & Klonoff, E. (1992). Culture and health-related schema's: A review and proposal for interdisciplinary integration. *Health Psychology, 11*, 267–276.

Lawton, M., Rajagopal, D., Brody, E., & Kleban, M. (1992). The dynamics of caregiving for a demented elder among Black and White families. *Journal of Gerontology: Social Sciences, 47*, 156–164.

Lazarus, R., & Folkman, S. (1984). Stress, appraisal, and coping. New York: Springer.

McLanahan, S., & Casper, L. (1995). Growing diversity and inequality in the American family. In R. Farley (Ed.), State of the union: America in the 1990s. Vol. 2: Social trends (pp. 1–45). New York: Sage.

Miller, B., Campbell, R., Farran, C., Kaufman, J., & Davis (1995). Race, control, mastery, and caregiver distress. *Journal of Gerontology: Social Sciences, 50*, 374–382.

Mills, P., Ziegler, M., Patterson, T., Dimsdale, J., Hauger, R., Irwin, M., & Grant, I. (1997). Plasma catecholine and lymphocyte beta-2 adrenergic receptor alterations in elderly Alzheimer's caregivers under stress. *Psychosomatic Medicine, 59*, 251–256.

Morycz, R., Malloy, J., Bozich, M., & Martz, P. (1987). Racial differences in family burden: Clinical implications for social work. In R. Dubroff (Ed.), Gerontological social work with families (pp. 133–154). New York: Haworth Press.

Mutran, E. (1985). Intergenerational family support among Blacks and Whites: Response to culture and socioeconomic differences. *Journal of Gerontology, 34*, 48–54.

Neighbors, H. (1997). Husbands, wives, familiy and friends: Sources of stress, sources of support. In R. Taylor, J. Jackson, & L. Chatters (Eds.), Family life in Black America (pp. 279–294). Thousand Oaks: Sage.

Nobles, W. (1980). African philosophy: Foundations for black psychology. In R. L. Jones (Ed.), *Black psychology* 2nd Edition. New York: Harper & Row.

Nobles, W. (1974). Africanity: It's role in Black families. *The Black Scholar*, 10–16.

Picot, S., Debanne, B., Namazi, K., & Wykle, M. (1997). Perceived rewards and religiosity among Black and White caregivers. *The Gerontologist, 37*, 612–619.

Schulz, R., O'Brien, D., Bookwalla, F., & Fleissner, J. (1995). Examining caregiver burden. *The Gerontologist, 35*, 181–191.

Skaff, M. (1995). Religion in the stress process: Coping with caregiving. Paper presented at the Annual Scientific Meeting of the Gerontological Society of America, Los Angeles, CA.

Taylor, R., Chatters, L., & Jackson, J. (Eds.). (1997). Family life in Black America. Thousand Oaks: Sage.

Taylor, R., Tucker, B., Chatters, L., & Jayakody. (1997). Recent demographic trends in African American family structure. In R. Taylor, J. Jackson, & L. Chatters (Eds.), Family life in Black America (pp. 14–62). Thousand Oaks: Sage.

U.S. Bureau of the Census. (1990). The need for personal assistance with everyday activities: Recipients and caregivers. Washington, DC: U.S. Government Office.

Vitaliano, P., Russo, J., Young, H., Teri, L., & Maiuro, R. (1991). Predictors of burden in spouse caregivers of individuals with Alzheimer's disease. *Psychology and Aging, 6*, 392–402.

Walls, C., & Zarit, S. (1991). Informal support from Black churches and the well-being of elderly Blacks. *The Gerontologist, 31,* 490–495.

Wheaton, B. (1985). Models of stress-buffering functions of coping resources. *Journal of Health and Social Behavior, 26,* 352–364.

Zarit, S., Reever, K., & Bach-Peterson, J. (1980). Relatives of impaired elderly: Correlates of feelings of burden. *The Gerontologist, 20,* 373–377.

Stress Level Monitoring

In this chapter, the foremost strategy of the Stress Reduction Technique—Stress Level Monitoring—is laid out. A description of stress and the cycle of distress is first provided, and following is the introduction of stress monitoring which includes the Daily Stress Rating (DSR) Form. There is a discussion of how to chart one's stress level, and the chapter closes with several case examples that demonstrate the use of this technique.

☐ Understanding Stress

The first step in introducing the strategies of the Stress Reduction Technique to caregivers is to provide an overview and basic definition of stress. It is important that this groundwork be laid for several reasons. First, the term *stress* is used differently by most people and it is a good starting place to make sure that there is general agreement about what, in fact, is being discussed and targeted. Second, caregivers will benefit from having a reference point throughout the learning process. Often, caregivers will have difficulty understanding how a particular strategy relates to the original problem of stress, and it is through this professional reminder of the basic description of stress that caregivers will be able to grasp the connection.

Different definitions of stress abound in the literature. Selye began writing about stress in the 1930s and has done extensive work on the stress process. Selye defined stress as "the nonspecific response of the body to any demand" (1980, p. 127) and his work has focused primarily on the body's physiological response to these demands. In the 1960s, Lazarus expanded the meaning of stress to include the environment and introduced the concepts of appraisal and coping. Lazarus and his colleague, Folkman defined psychological stress as "a relationship between the person and the environment that is appraised by the person as taxing or exceeding his or her resources and endangering his or her well-being" (1984, p. 19). This definition moved beyond Selye's tradition that stress is a singular response (Hobfoll, 1988). Within the Lazarus model, *appraisal* is the process by which a person assesses the stressfulness of a situation or circumstance (Holroyd & Lazarus, 1982; Lazarus, 1966). And *coping* is a person's efforts to manage both environmental and internal demands as well as conflicts between demands (Holroyd & Lazarus, 1982; Lazarus, 1966).

A definition of stress that has been widely used by stress researchers is that of McGrath (Hobfoll, 1988). He defined stress as a "substantial imbalance between environmental demand and the response capability of the focal organism" (McGrath, 1970, p. 17). McGrath proposed that *imbalance* is based on subjective perceptions, and *demand* involves quantitative and qualitative properties. An additional definition of stress was offered by Kaplan who stated that psychological stress "reflects the subject's inability to forestall or diminish perception, recall, anticipation, or imagination of disvalued circumstances, those that in reality or fantasy signify great and/or increased distance from desirable (valued) experiential states, and consequently, evoke a need to approximate the valued states" (Kaplan, 1983, p. 196). Hobfoll combined Kaplan's and McGrath's definitions to suggest that "stress is the state in which individuals judge their response capabilities as unable to meet the threat to the loss of desirable experiential states—states that are dictated by their values and expectations" (Hobfoll, 1988, p. 19).

This is a small sampling of some of the definitions of stress that exist and, clearly, there are countless others. Although there are many ways to view the term *stress*, it generally is acknowledged that stress involves not only a stressor, but also an individual's appraisal of the stressor. In working with caregivers, a very basic definition of stress serves useful: Stress is a response to change. This simple and concise statement is effective because it allows caregivers to understand that stress can be either positive or negative, and it also suggests that, although caregivers may not be able to control the caregiving situation, they can control their reaction to change. It is caregivers' awareness both of this reaction and of their ability to impact the appraisal process that is critical in order for them to believe they can affect their stress level.

Stress can be positive, on one hand, because it can be a motivating factor that stimulates better performance and accomplishments. For example, the change in an older relative's ambulation abilities may motivate the caregiver to take the relative to a physician, resulting in physical therapy to help the relative walk better. This result allows the caregiver to feel successful in this role, satisfied that he or she is helping to keep the relative's quality of life as high as possible, and also reduces the amount of physical care that the caregiver has to provide.

On the other hand, negative stress is a response to a change that yields no constructive outcome. For example, the day-to-day stressors of caregiving, such as when the relative continually is obstinate about personal care tasks, can add up and become overwhelming for the caregiver. A negative response would occur if the caregiver does nothing to try to counterbalance the stress and merely becomes more and more frustrated. This emotional reaction to negative stress can be described as distress. *Distress* implies mental strain imposed by emotional pain, worry, or constant demands. Often, distress is manifested as fear, anger, frustration, and anxiety. If the demands or stressors are continual, distress often can evolve into depression or anxiety disorders such as phobias. Physical responses can include increased blood pressure and heart rate, muscle tension, dizziness due to an increase in rate of breathing, and an increase in perspiration.

Prolonged stress can affect both physical and emotional health. Negative stress that is extended or frequent can wear on the entire body and eventually can cause permanent damage and disease. For example, increased blood pressure, when perpetuated, can cause cardiovascular disorders such as heart attack or stroke. Ongoing stomach tension as a result of stress is related to gastrointestinal problems, and constant muscle tension can lead to chronic fatigue, headaches, backaches, and muscle pain. Research indicates that stress is related to many different illnesses including gastrointestinal disorders, cardiovascular disease, atherosclerosis, hypertension, cancer, endocrine disease, hyperthyroidism, pulmonary disease, bronchial asthma, chronic obstructive pulmonary disease, and hematological disease (Bunney et al., 1982). Furthermore, stress is believed to impact the entire body's immune system, making a person more vulnerable to illness (Minter & Kimball, 1980). According to Zegans, "There appears to be anatomical, physiological, and neurochemical evidence that cognitive-affective responses to stress can alter the functioning of those vital hypothalamic-pituitary pathways that modulate endocrine, autonomic, and immune processes. Alteration of these systems and of the brain sets the stage for the onset of disease" (1982, p. 150).

Ongoing stress also can have an impact on emotional health. Unrelenting distress can lead to a variety of emotional reactions, including depression, anxiety, and frustration. Mrs. Strickland is an 80-year-old African American woman who has been caring for her husband for the past 8 years. He recently became incontinent. When asked to describe some emotional reactions she had to this added stressor, she broke down in tears and replied,

"I guess I don't have to tell you what my emotional reaction is." Further discussion with Mrs. Strickland resulted in her sharing that she cries every day, but has gotten used to it; it has become a normal way of living. With long-term stress, these emotional reactions may last a long time. Caregivers may become used to these distressing emotions and come to consider them as normal and usual feelings, whereas these emotions would have been recognized as problems in less stressful times.

Given the potential impact of ongoing distress on the caregiver's health, it is important to begin to explore various means of helping the caregiver reduce this stress once a general understanding of stress is established. The first strategy of Stress Level Monitoring takes caregivers' understanding of stress to another level, allowing them to personalize the stress that they are experiencing. It is the first step in the Stress Reduction Technique and it will help caregivers determine when stress reduction strategies are needed.

☐ The Cycle of Distress

For caregivers, there will be moments when they feel relaxed for one reason or another, and times when they will feel distressed. If they do not deal with the stress when they first experience it, it likely will become a vicious cycle and develop into a pattern that maintains or heightens their stress level. For example, caregivers may feel distress over lack of family support. This distress may be manifested as anger or lashing out at a family member. Caregivers may then develop feelings of guilt over their behavior, thereby compounding their feelings of distress. In the case of Ms. Strickland, although she considered daily crying as normal, she complained about her daughter and son who rarely came to visit. When they did come, the visit inevitably would end up in an argument after which they would leave. Afterward she would feel guilty for starting the argument, and would feel even more distressed about her caregiving situation. When caregivers experience distress on a continual basis without any relief, they place themselves at increased risk of emotional health problems, as with Ms. Strickland, and also physical health problems. Therefore, it is important that caregivers have a daily awareness of where they are in the cycle.

Every person experiences stress differently; hence, it is important for caregivers to have a baseline of what is stressful for them while trying to determine where they are in the cycle of distress. For example, one caregiver may find a day full of doctors' appointments very distressing, while another caregiver may not. Furthermore, it is not merely the events that may cause stress for caregivers, but also what else is going on in their life on a particular day.

☐ The Use of Monitoring

An important way for caregivers to understand their baseline or average level of stress and also assess where they are in the cycle of distress is to begin monitoring their stress level on a daily basis. This concept has been used by Lewinsohn, Munoz, Youngren, and Zeiss (1992, p. 38) in treating depression. Lewinsohn's approach is that, by tracking one's level of mood, one is able to evaluate how successful one is at improving it. It is used as a tool in helping a person "look carefully at her activities and interactions to determine which activities lead to positive outcomes and which activities are associated with negative outcomes." Also, it allows people to increase awareness of the impact of events on their mood. Likewise, this same approach can be applied to managing stress. All caregivers have stress, and it is important to first have caregivers describe some of the stress they are experiencing. The professional can write down the stress as the caregivers describe it and keep it for reviewing in later discussions. This will help to individualize the program and serve as a reference later when introducing the DSR (discussed below).

In order to help caregivers grasp the role of monitoring their stress level, the following three points should be kept in mind. First, it is critical that they learn to recognize exactly when they feel distressed. What situations are occurring when they have these negative feelings? They should be reminded that both positive and negative situations can cause them to feel distressed. For example, they may feel distressed at a family gathering (a positive situation) because of fear of how other relatives may react to the behavior of the person with dementia. Or, they may feel distressed when their relative begins to wander from home (a negative situation).

Second, caregivers should learn to identify what specifically about a situation makes them feel calm and what makes them feel distressed. Often there are good and bad components to an event, so caregivers need to determine what about a situation helps them feel calm and minimizes distress, and then focus on maximizing these positive aspects. For example, when caregivers are taking their spouse to the doctor, they may find that if they allow plenty of time and first stop to eat at a restaurant, their spouse is better adjusted by the time they reach the doctor's office. On the other hand, if caregivers do not allow enough time and have to rush to make the appointment, their spouse may become more irritable and therefore cause the caregivers to feel distressed. Realizing this, caregivers can allow for extra time on their next visit to the doctor, which will help them to feel less stressed.

Third, in addition to recognizing when caregivers feel distressed and what causes the distress, caregivers should learn to ascertain where they are in the distress cycle. It is important for caregivers to not generalize their position. Few people are highly stressed all of the time. Most people have "good" and "bad" days. It may be useful to have caregivers compare their present position in the cycle to those times when they have felt more or less distress, in order to accurately perceive where they now are in the cycle. Once caregivers recognize these three basic ideas—the when, the what, and the where of the distress cycle—they are ready to be introduced to the DSR form.

☐ The Daily Stress Rating Form

Although few people are highly stressed all the time, most people fail to recognize this and feel that they are constantly under stress. The DSR form provides a method of tracking the caregiver's stress level in order to demonstrate that there truly are "good" days and "bad" days. It also provides the first step toward changing the caregiver's stress level: identifying when the stress happens.

The DSR is fairly easy to understand. It includes a scale that is meant to be a numeric representation of the overall stress level for each day, ranging from "very calm" (9) to "very distressed" (1). The idea is for caregivers to take 2 to 3 minutes at the end of the day to reflect on the events that took place, compare and contrast their images of calm events and distressing ones in a nondetailed manner, and then record an overall impression of the day on the DSR sheet. Figure 3-1 gives a sample of the DSR form.

The caregiver should be aware that few people have a day that is a 9, which might be compared to feeling as if one is basking in the sun on a deserted island. Likewise, few people are on the other end of the scale with a 1, feeling as if everything that could go wrong did, and are completely overwhelmed. The purpose of this form is that, by having caregivers look at their daily stress level, they will avoid generalizing and saying that they have nothing but stressful days. Instead, caregivers will recognize that days, like feelings, are different. It also is hoped that caregivers will realize that they have some days that actually are good.

By allowing caregivers to look back on the events and feelings of the day, the DSR can show caregivers that their feelings affect their stress level. It highlights the connection between the events of the day, the caregivers' behavior or reactions to those events, and their overall distress level. The key to understanding this connection is knowing what is happening at the time caregivers are having these distressing feelings.

After explaining the process to the caregivers, it is useful for the professional to go through an example. The professional should give the caregivers a copy of the DSR and have them rate the day's distress feelings. Then the

Please rate your level of stress for this day, i.e. how calm or distressed you feel, using the nine-point scale shown below. Enter the date in column 2 and your stress score in column 3. If you felt really calm (the best you have ever felt or can imagine yourself feeling), mark 9. If you felt really distressed (the worst you have ever felt or can imagine yourself feeling), mark 1. If it was a "so-so" (or mixed) day, mark 5. If you felt worse than "so-so," mark a number between 2 and 4. If you felt better than "so-so," mark a number between 6 and 8. **Remember, a low number signifies that you felt distressed, and a high number means that you felt calm today.**

Very Distressed 1   2   3   4   5   6   7   8   9   **Very Calm**

Monitoring Day	Date	Stress Score	Monitoring Day	Date	Stress Score	Monitoring Day	Date	Stress Score
1			16			31		
2			17			32		
3			18			33		
4			19			34		
5			20			35		
6			21			36		
7			22			37		
8			23			38		
9			24			39		
10			25			40		
11			26			41		
12			27			42		
13			28			43		
14			29			44		
15			30			45		

FIGURE 3-1. Daily Stress Rating (DSR) form.

professional should help the caregivers fill out the form, and offer feedback to the caregivers on how they have used the form. The caregivers should be given the form to use for several days, and may need help from the professional to work toward using it independently.

The Use of Charting

Once the caregivers have become familiar and comfortable with using the DSR form, helping them chart their stress level for a week at a time will enhance their ability to monitor their stress level. They should be able

The scale provided is meant to be a numeric representation of the day overall, ranging from "very calm" (9) to "very distressed" (1). The idea is for you to take two to three minutes at the end of the day to reflect on the events that took place. Compare and contrast your images of calm events and distressing ones in a non-detailed manner, then record an overall impression of the day and the date on the sheet.

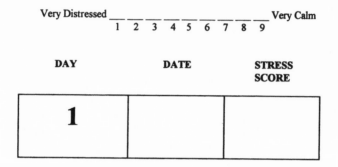

- Take 2 to 3 minutes to reflect on the day.
- Compare and contrast events of the day.
- Record the number that correlates with your overall impression.

FIGURE 3-1. Daily Stress Rating (DSR) form (continued).

to determine what their personal average distress level is by averaging their previous stress scores on the DSR; this can be used as a baseline for measuring where their stress level is in any given week. A caregiver's chart may look like Figure 3-2 for one week.

Note that the level of distress fluctuates from day to day; some days are less stressful than others, which is to be expected. It may be helpful for

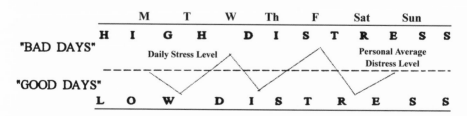

FIGURE 3-2. Example of a caregiver's charted stress level for one week.

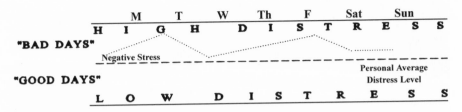

FIGURE 3-3. Example of a caregiver's charted stress that may indicate a negative stress level.

caregivers to think of the ups and downs in terms of "good" days and "bad" days. Another chart for the same caregiver in a different week may look like Figure 3-3.

Note that, during this second week, the caregiver continually stays above his or her personal average distress level (Figure 3-3). This often is an indication that the caregiver's stress level has become negative and potentially can be harmful if the caregiver does not seek ways to intervene in the cycle. Appropriate use of interventions at this point can change the direction of the spiral of increasing stress. Hence, charting can allow caregivers to visualize both their average daily stress level and if they are deviating from that average.

☐ Case Examples

Generally speaking, this first strategy is readily embraced by caregivers. It is easy for most caregivers to grasp, and most important, it takes very little time and thought. The challenge, however, is to help caregivers maintain continual use of this strategy and utilize it as a tool to indicate the need for further interventions. The following cases demonstrate this more fully.

Mr. Ramos

Mr. Ramos is a single man in his early forties. He has been caring for his mother, who has dementia, since the death of his father in 1985. A man who considers himself a natural to the role of caregiving, Mr. Ramos has accepted caregiving as his familial obligation, despite the stress that comes from providing care and the loss of personal freedom.

Mr. Ramos's caregiving role actually began before the death of his father, who soon after retirement began displaying symptoms of Parkinson's disease. Then, his father suffered a stroke and became even more functionally impaired. Mr. Ramos's mother became the primary caregiver for her long-time spouse, and Mr. Ramos became his mother's support. As he observed the amount of stress his mother was under, he shifted more and more into supporting and caring for her. Before his father's death, as Mr. Ramos gradually became more involved, his mother began demonstrating symptoms of dementia. She began to require assistance, and her son was "the obvious" caregiver.

There was a strong sense of reciprocity between Mr. Ramos and his parents, and this was especially true with his mother, to whom he was always close. When he was growing up, his mother seemed depressed, particularly in the 1960s when she was a "stereotypical housewife." Whereas his brother seemed to "block everything out," as a child Mr. Ramos felt his mother's depression and did his best to help her feel better. He also tried to make up for the fact that his father worked long hours while his mother was alone at home.

In spite of the fact that Mr. Ramos felt that being a caregiver was the right thing to do, he inevitably experienced a lot of stress from the role. First, his work was a source of distress. Mr. Ramos had a high-pressure job during the first few years of his mother's illness, and it increasingly became impossible for him to perform well in addition to giving her adequate care. His mother constantly would call him while he was at work, and he had difficulty concentrating. When it reached a point of culmination, he made the difficult decision to leave his job and move in with his mother to become her full-time caregiver. Although Mr. Ramos feels good about this decision, it is a constant source of worry because he wonders about the future of his career, and when and if he should reenter the workforce.

Second, Mr. Ramos finds that trying to access resources for his mother is a constant source of stress. He will not consider placing his mother in a nursing home, as he promised long ago never to do this. He has found adult day care centers unfriendly to him as a caregiver due to their limited hours and inability to handle his mother's behavioral problems like resistance and agitation. Cost also is an issue for Mr. Ramos, and he feels strongly that professionals do not recognize the reality of this factor when recommending respite.

Third, Mr. Ramos has had great difficulty maintaining personal relationships while being a caregiver. His friends do not seem willing to understand his position, and he looks to them mainly for occasional social interaction. Also, while being a caregiver, he started a relationship with a woman, but became unable to continue it because she wanted to talk about their future and Mr. Ramos could not consider giving up his role as caregiver.

When Mr. Ramos began to learn the Stress Reduction Technique, he was under a great deal of stress which was manifesting itself in both physical and emotional symptoms. He had great difficulty distinguishing between what aspects of his role were stressful and what aspects were not; to him, it was entirely stressful all of the time. When the concept of Stress Level Monitoring was introduced to Mr. Ramos, he thought it would be easy to do, and was convinced that he would be rating every day a 1. Due to his busy daily schedule and the fact that he rarely had a minute to himself, it was necessary to strategize with him as to when he would use the DSR form in order to ensure that it would be used every day. After going through in detail how Mr. Ramos spent his days, he agreed that the best time to try to use the form was after dinner, when his mother usually was content to watch television for 30 minutes.

After trying the DSR form for 1 week, Mr. Ramos reported that it was not what he had expected. While he agreed that it was very easy to use, he was having difficulty remembering to use it daily, and finding time for it at the end of the day. On this particular week, his mother had been increasingly agitated after dinner and Mr. Ramos found that he could not leave her unattended. By the time he got his mother to bed, he had forgotten about the form and was so exhausted he collapsed into bed. Also, Mr. Ramos indicated that he had a hard time determining where he fell on the scale. He did indeed feel that every day had been a 1.

Further discussion and problem solving resulted in a different plan for Mr. Ramos on week 2. Mr. Ramos agreed that he would leave the form on his bedside stand under his alarm clock, and try to use it every morning when he awoke to record a score for the previous day. He was able to recognize that mornings were generally calmer regardless of his mother's agitation level, as she usually needed to be awakened by Mr. Ramos and he typically had some time to himself before doing this. Trying to help him comprehend the DSR scale was a little more challenging. Considerable time was spent going over examples and then asking Mr. Ramos to recall a day where he felt less stressed than he had during the past week. It was necessary for Mr. Ramos to recall a day several months previous, but eventually he was able to agree that on that day he felt less stressed than he had been during the previous week. Using this as a reference, Mr. Ramos was then able to utilize the DSR scale and reflect on the prior week, resulting in a different score for each day. As a result of helping Mr. Ramos identify a better time to try to record his daily stress level, and assisting him in understanding how to apply the scale, Mr. Ramos was willing to continue using the DSR for a second week.

Following the second week, Mr. Ramos reported that he was successful in utilizing the form, and that it made more sense to him. Since he had 1 full week of scores, the next step was to chart his week in order to help him visualize his stress level. This proved to be very useful for Mr. Ramos, as he was able to identify that the middle of the week was most stressful for him. He recalled the events of the middle of the week and was able to ascertain what about the situation was distressing. From this, he was able to consider ways to help alleviate his stress should the situation occur.

Mr. Ramos continued to utilize the DSR form and charting to learn more about his stress. It became a very simple and quick way for him to be in touch with how he was managing, and it slowly diminished his tendency to catastrophize how stressful his role was. It also allowed him to move on and learn the other strategies in the Stress Reduction Technique.

Ms. Duncan

Ms. Duncan is a middle-aged woman who has been caring for her mother for many years. It all started when her father was diagnosed with cancer and had surgery. Ms. Duncan's parents were living in Texas and, following her father's surgery, she temporarily moved to Texas to help out. During this time, she noticed that her mother also was declining. After an evaluation, her mother was diagnosed with Alzheimer's disease. Ms. Duncan moved to southern California and decided to bring both parents along to live with her. Her father recovered from the surgery, but her mother continued to deteriorate cognitively.

Ms. Duncan reflects that she always has been a loving person and, as a child, she cared for her grandmother. She sees herself as a "people pleaser," which explains why she decided to care for her parents when her older sister claimed she was too busy and her brother asserted that he could not impose on his wife. Ms. Duncan reports that she saw a need and stepped in; there was no other way to handle the situation. It was clear that her mother could not help care for father during his recovery, and neither could her father help her mother. So, Ms. Duncan moved her parents into the small mobile home where she and her husband resided.

What developed in the following years was not easy. Ms. Duncan's husband was not supportive of her decision to move both parents into their small home, and this became a great source of contention in their marriage. Ms. Duncan often felt angry not only because she lacked her husband's support, but also because it was a constant source of conflict between them. After several years of their being unable to resolve this conflict, Ms. Duncan's husband left her and moved to Washington.

Ms. Duncan recognized that her home was a difficult environment to live in. Her mother constantly was wandering around the small space, seemingly in circles and agitated, and her father could not accept that it was a disease and that her mother could not control her behavior. In addition, although Ms. Duncan had lived apart from her parents for many years, her father seemed to slip back into his previous role of father once they moved in together. He expected Ms. Duncan to wait on him constantly, and he frequently voiced his opinion and disapproval of her daily activities. Once her husband left, her father seemed to constantly vacillate on how terrible that was. Ms. Duncan increasingly felt frustrated at the fact that her home was no longer hers, but continued to feel the need to provide the care she was giving.

Ms. Duncan worked at a private religious school nearby, and frequently had to leave during the workday to help with a crisis such as her mother leaving the home and her father being unable to manage the situation. There also were constant phone calls and she often found it hard to concentrate. However, in spite of the stressors that seemed to impede her work life, Ms. Duncan also reported that it has been her coworkers and friends at her church who provided the greatest support to her during the most trying days.

As her mother's condition progressively worsened, Ms. Duncan came to the difficult realization that she could no longer keep her at home. Along with the increased agitation, memory loss, and confusion, her mother was starting to fall frequently. Her father had hernia surgery and was unable to provide the hands-on care that Ms. Duncan's mother was beginning to require. Ms. Duncan could not quit her job as this was her only source of income. So, with the encouragement of her friends, she made the decision to place her mother in a nursing home. This was one of the most difficult and painful parts of being a caregiver, according to Ms. Duncan. Once she went through this troublesome process and got to the place where she was able to limit her visits to the nursing home, she began to rebuild her life. However, her father still continued to live with her and she resented how this was holding her back from moving on.

It was during the demanding stage of her mother's worsening health that Ms. Duncan was introduced to the Stress Reduction Technique. She was enthusiastic about trying the strategies because she felt she would collapse unless she got some help in dealing with the situation. When the DSR form was introduced to Ms. Duncan, she was anxious to begin to understand more about her stress level. She decided that she would try to fill out the form at the end of the day after dinner, as she usually had some time to sit down and relax once the dishes were done.

After the first week, Ms. Duncan was surprised that, although it seemed easy to sit down and rate her day, she had difficulty doing it consistently every day. She had failed to realize that 2 days a week she had to rush to activities at her church following dinner. And, on the nights that she was at home, her mother's increasing agitation in the evening made it difficult for her to find time after the dishes were done. Also, her stress level often went up after she had rated her day, because getting her mother to follow through with personal hygiene tasks before bedtime was becoming more challenging. Following some discussion, Ms. Duncan decided that a better approach would be to fill out the form as part of her own bedtime routine. Ms. Duncan seemed to understand how to rate her stress level, but she just had not been able to do it for more than 3 days that week. Ms. Duncan was determined to complete all 7 days for the second week.

After the second week, Ms. Duncan did indeed find that the later time worked better for her in recording her stress level. She had managed to rate her stress level for 7 days, and the next step was to help her chart the week. Once this was done and she could look at a visual representation of the week, Ms. Duncan was very surprised that she rated her stress level as high for only 3 out of the 7 days. When asked how her week went, she had responded that it was very stressful. On further discussion, however, Ms. Duncan was able to realize that it was not that every day was stressful, but it was that the amount of stress she experienced on 3 of the days was so high. She recalled the events of those 3 days and was able to identify particular situations that were very distressing. For example, when her mother refused to eat at the dinner table, it not only was the frustration of trying to coerce her into eating that was disturbing, but also her father's yelling at her mother was particularly upsetting. Ms. Duncan was able to gain a new perspective on specifically what caused her to feel distressed, and to use this information when she learned the additional strategies of the technique. For example, she was able to recognize that, when dinner was particularly disturbing, she needed to utilize a strategy to help bring her stress level down before trying to go to sleep. Once Ms. Duncan was able to make the connection between rating, charting, and taking steps to reduce her stress, she was convinced that this was the only way to manage on a daily basis and continued to use the DSR throughout her entire caregiving career.

☐ Summary

Helping caregivers understand stress and begin to utilize Stress Level Monitoring is the first step in introducing the Stress Reduction Technique. It is critical that enough time be spent at this early stage to help caregivers grasp the reason for and use of this basic tool in order for the remaining strategies to be effective. Unless caregivers can be empowered to recognize when they feel distressed, what specifically about the situation makes them feel calm and what makes them feel distressed, and where they are in the distress cycle, they will have great difficulty taking the next step to reduce their stress. However, if caregivers can master these steps with the use of the DSR form and weekly charting, they will be able to learn the additional strategies central to the technique and move forward in alleviating their distress.

☐ References

Hobfoll, S. E. (1988). *The ecology of stress*. New York: Hemisphere.

Holroyd, K. A., & Lazarus, R. S. (1982). Stress, coping, and somatic adaptation. In L. Goldberger & S. Brezniz (Eds.), *Handbook of stress: Theoretical and clinical aspects* (pp. 21–35). New York: The Free Press.

Kaplan, H. B. (1983). Psychological distress in sociological context: Toward a general theory of psychosocial stress. In H. B. Kaplan (Ed.), *Psychosocial stress: Trends in theory and research* (pp. 195–264). New York: Academic Press.

Lazarus, R. S. (1966). *Psychological stress and the coping process*. New York: McGraw-Hill.

Lazarus, R. S., & Folkman, S. (1984). *Stress, appraisal, and coping*. New York: Springer.

Lewinsohn, P. M., Munoz, R. F., Youngren, M., & Zeiss, A. M. (1992). *Control your depression*. New York: Fireside, Simon & Shuster.

McGrath, J. E. (1970). A conceptual formulation for research on stress. In J. E. McGrath (Ed.), *Social and psychological factors in stress* (pp. 10–21). New York: Holt, Rinehart & Winston.

Minter, R. E., & Kimball, C. P. (1980). Life events, personality traits, and illness. In I. L. Kutash, L. B. Schlesinger & Associates (Eds.), *Handbook on stress and anxiety: Contemporary knowledge, theory, and treatment* (pp. 189–206). San Francisco: Jossey-Bass.

Selye, H. (1980). The stress concept today. In I. L. Kutash, L. B. Schlesinger & Associates (Eds.), *Handbook on stress and anxiety: Contemporary knowledge, theory, and treatment* (pp. 127–143). San Francisco: Jossey-Bass.

Zegans, L. S. (1982). Stress and the development of somatic disorders. In L. Goldberger & S. Brezniz (Eds.), *Handbook of stress: Theoretical and clinical aspects* (pp. 134–152). New York: The Free Press.

CHAPTER

Progressive Relaxation and Visualization

An important aspect of assisting caregivers in managing their stress is helping them recognize the usefulness of strategies that can reduce the symptoms of stress. In this chapter, two tools that are useful for caregivers to learn will be presented: progressive relaxation and visualization. A short review and history of progressive relaxation will be presented, and then each strategy will be described. Also included are instructions for progressive relaxation and visualization which can be used with caregivers. As with chapter 3, this chapter will conclude with three case studies.

☐ Progressive Relaxation

Progressive relaxation is unique to the many other existing forms of relaxation in that it requires muscle tension release cycles. The actual term *progressive relaxation* was coined in 1929 by Jacobson, and was used to describe a method that "could quiet the nerve-muscle system, including what is commonly called the 'mind'" (Jacobson, 1929; 1957, p. 87). Jacobson proposed that, even when one lies on a couch and tries to relax, there still remains "residual tension" that can dissipate only through concentrated relaxation of each part of the body. In effect, he suggested that, if one could relax the muscles, inevitably one could then relax mentally; the more relaxed the muscles, the more relaxed one would feel inside (Woolfolk &

Richardson, 1979). In its original form as developed by Jacobson, progressive relaxation could involve as much as 40 individual sessions, covering nearly 30 to 39 muscle groups (Carlson & Hoyle, 1993; Jacobson, 1929; Woolfolk & Richardson, 1979). In 1973, Bernstein and Borkovec produced a more abbreviated form of the technique in a manual which involves 8 to 12 sessions, covering 16 muscle groups. This streamlined version of the technique has allowed it to be greatly utilized by clinicians.

Many studies have been performed to evaluate the effectiveness of progressive relaxation in treating various physiological and psychological disorders. A quantitative review of research studies between 1981 and 1992 that used Bernstein and Borkovec's abbreviated progressive relaxation training (ABRT) was undertaken by Carlson and Hoyle (1993). They concluded that, on the whole, ABRT has been found to be an effective treatment for a range of disorders, including tension headaches, hypertension, cancer, and psychophysiological disorders, often involving pain management. Several studies also have been done on the effects of progressive relaxation in reducing insomnia in older adults (Engle-Friedman, Hazlewood, Bootzin, & Tsao, 1992; Gustafson, 1992; Piercy & Lohr, 1989), demonstrating that it is a useful form of treatment. However, it also has been noted that, for some older adults, progressive relaxation can be ineffective because of physical limitations that contraindicate muscle tension release procedures (Scogin, Rickard, Keith, Wilson, & McElreath, 1992). Scogin et al. (1992) suggested that imaginal relaxation, which requires passive focusing on physiological sensations, is a beneficial alternate option for those older adults unable to engage in progressive relaxation—in particular, older adults experiencing anxiety-related symptoms. Progressive relaxation, then, appears to be an effective tool for treating various stress-related symptoms, with the exception of older adults who may have chronic conditions which preclude them from using the technique. For these older adults, a similar exercise can be used, but they should be instructed to imagine these operations as opposed to actually tensing the muscles.

For caregivers, progressive relaxation can help them become aware of and control various muscles that may become tense and contribute to stress. Also, when caregivers are relaxed, they are less likely to become anxious and depressed. Learning to relax is similar to learning a skill and, with regular practice, caregivers can control their bodily tension and experience a greater degree of relaxation more of the time. It is recommended that caregivers practice progressive relaxation from 10 to 20 minutes, at least once a day. They should not worry if their progress seems slow. As long as caregivers work at the procedure and practice conscientiously, they will gradually experience an enjoyable state of relaxation. The key is to not try too hard and to not rush through the relaxation exercises.

Some common problems that caregivers may experience when doing relaxation therapy include external distractions, distracting thoughts, and physical reactions. First, external distractions can be avoided by encouraging caregivers to carefully select a time and place where they will not be disturbed. This may be very difficult given the constant attention that care recipients may require. It should be suggested that caregivers come up with creative times and places to perform the exercise. Some examples that caregivers may try include waking up 30 minutes before the care recipient wakes, performing the technique after the care recipient is asleep, trying to occupy the care recipient with an independent task (i.e., folding clothes), or suggesting that the care recipient take a short nap. After a while, caregivers will be less and less disturbed by minor distractions, such as worrying about the care recipient or hearing the care recipient in the other room. Second, caregivers' minds may wander during practice sessions and they may be plagued by distracting thoughts. This is common for people under a great deal of stress, so they should not become discouraged. Instead, caregivers should try to redirect their attention to their breathing or to relaxing their muscles. Third, at times, caregivers may experience small muscle spasms, jerks, or tingling sensations while they relax. These physical reactions actually are signs that they are relaxing and, with further practice, these reactions will decrease or become so familiar that they no longer will be distracting. These three common difficulties should be addressed and explained to caregivers before starting the technique, to ensure that, if they occur, caregivers will not automatically abandon the method.

Progressive relaxation consists of tensing and relaxing various muscles, and slow deep breathing. The muscle tensing and relaxing occurs in five steps. First, caregivers turn their attention to the muscles to be relaxed. Second, they tense the muscles, not so that it hurts, but enough so that they can feel the tension. If caregivers happen to have chronic pain in any part of their body, they should not tense these parts. As suggested by Scogin et al. (1992), caregivers should be instructed to use imaginal relaxation if chronic pain is experienced during the tensing of muscles, whether this be for particular muscles or for the entire exercise. For example, if caregivers have arthritis in their wrists, they may wish to utilize progressive relaxation techniques in other muscle groups of their bodies but, when they relax their arms and hands, they should use imaginal relaxation and simply imagine the relaxing of these muscles. Third, caregivers gradually let the tension go and feel the muscles unwind. Fourth, they tense the muscles again, but not as much as before. Last, caregivers gradually let the tension go and feel the muscles unwind completely. Slow deep breathing, which occurs in conjunction with the muscle relaxation, involves inhaling, holding the breath briefly, and then slowly letting out one's breath between slightly parted lips. As one breathes out, it is important to also let the tension go. These two techniques are essential for caregivers to learn, in order for progressive relaxation to be effective.

It is important for caregivers to realize that relaxation is a skill and, therefore, it may not work for them the first time they try it. But, with practice, caregivers can learn how to gain control over their muscle tension and begin to enjoy the feelings of relaxation. After caregivers have learned the technique, they can experience it on their own whenever they feel distressed.

Instructions

The following is a script that the professional can use with caregivers for progressive relaxation. The professional should take care to move very slowly and methodically through the exercise, making sure to pause after each step. The exercise should take at least 20 minutes, and every effort should be made to make sure caregivers are in a quiet place, free from distractions. It may be helpful to play soft music if noise distractions cannot be minimized.

Caregivers should be encouraged to follow each instruction carefully, even though it may seem uncomfortable at first. The purpose of going through the exercise with caregivers is to allow them to experience it and therefore increase the possibility that they will continue to use the technique regularly. If possible, the professional should go through the relaxation exercise with caregivers on a weekly basis for several weeks. The exercise goes as follows:

> Settle back as comfortably as you can. Let yourself relax to the best of your ability. Now, close your eyes. Take a few deep breaths. Inhale. Exhale. Inhale. Feel the tension building as you inhale. Exhale. Feel the tension leaving your body as you exhale; all the tensions of the day are going out of your body. Inhale once again. Hold your breath. Exhale.
>
> I'm going to ask you to tense each muscle two times. The first time, tense quite hard; the second time, only half as much. Now, let us begin.
>
> Tighten your feet muscles. Hold it, relax. Experience the sensation of relaxation when you relax your feet. As you feel the tension leaving your feet, allow this soothing feeling to move upward to your ankles. Repeat.
>
> To relax your calf muscles, press your feet and toes downward, away from your face, so your calf muscles become tense. Hold for a few seconds, then relax. Repeat once again. This time, bend your feet toward your face so that you feel tension along your shins. Bring your toes right up. Relax again. The second time, tense half as much.
>
> Tighten the muscles in your thighs by pushing them against the chair. Hold. Relax. Once again.

Tighten your buttocks muscles. Hold. Release. Again. Hold. Relax.

Pull the muscles of your stomach inward. Try to visualize your navel pressing against your spine and organs inside. I seem to hold a lot of tension in my stomach; maybe you do, too. I like to think of all my organs as rubber bands. Hold. Relax. The second time only half as hard. Tense. Release.

Next, you are going to relax your shoulders and upper back. You have two choices: Pull your shoulders back as though you were trying to touch your shoulder blades together, or you may want to try an alternate movement by raising your shoulders as though you were trying to touch your ears with the tops of your shoulders. Hold. Release. Repeat once again.

Hold your arms out and make a fist. Hold. Release. Repeat, the second time half as hard. Relax.

For the neck, there are two techniques to choose from. Pull your chin toward your chest using the muscles in the front of your neck, or you may wish to pull your head back with the muscles pushing back toward the wall. Begin tensing your muscles. Hold. Relax. Experience the relaxation for a brief period of time, then repeat.

Clench your teeth and pull back the corners of your mouth. At the same time, press your tongue firmly against the roof of your mouth. Hold. Release. Repeat once again.

Make a face. Raise your eyebrows as high as they will go. Wrinkle your brows and nose. Shut your eyelids tightly together. Hold for several seconds. Relax. Repeat again.

Now as you sit in your chair, with eyes closed, explore each of the regions you have relaxed. Think about your feet, calves and shins, thighs, buttocks, stomach, upper back, shoulders, arms, neck, mouth, and face. Try to be aware of any tension left in these muscles. If you are now free from tension, just quietly savor the feelings of calmness and relaxation. (Adapted from Woolfolk & Richardson, 1979, pp. 152–155).

☐ Visualization

Visualization is a technique that should follow the progressive relaxation exercise, but it also can be done on its own. It involves creating an image in one's mind that is tranquil and restful, and allowing oneself to be in that place for a period. Visualization allows one to imagine relaxation spreading through one's body. It enables one to escape a stressful environment for a brief duration, visit a very serene place, and then return to the stressful environment refreshed and with more energy. There is little empirical research available to demonstrate the effectiveness of visualization, but it is a technique that seems to be part of most current popular stress reduction material and it often is practiced in cancer and pain centers. Visualization is a particularly useful tool to use with caregivers because often caregivers are surrounded by stressors.

Instructions

The following is a script the professional can use with caregivers as a visualization exercise. It should follow the progressive relaxation technique for optimum effectiveness. As is true with progressive relaxation, the professional should take care to move very slowly and methodically through the exercise, making sure to pause after each statement. Caregivers should be encouraged to form mental sense impressions and involve all of their senses. This exercise should take an additional 10 to 15 minutes.

> Now, I want you to picture a blank screen in your mind. It may look like a TV or movie screen. Now, that you have the screen in mind, I want you to start with a dot of color in the middle of it. Choose a color that you find relaxing. For some people, that color may be yellow, blue, or orange. Choose any color that you find soothing. Now, let that color fill your screen. Once you have the color filling the screen, we will paint a picture on the screen. Now that you are relaxed, imagine yourself in a calm and peaceful place. Continue to take deep breaths. As your breathing gets deeper and slower, take yourself to a favorite spot. You may picture yourself in the mountains, at the beach, or in any tranquil environment that you like. This is a place just for you. It is warm, timeless, and tranquil. Your breathing is long and slow. There is no tension in your body and your mind is calm and relaxed. You feel at peace with yourself and fully relaxed. Your breathing is slow, deep, and steady, and you are enjoying your state of being. This is a time just for you. You are safe, calm, and warm. Time has disappeared and you may find yourself drifting. You continue to breathe slowly and enjoy your state of deep relaxation.
>
> When you are ready, slowly begin to ease back into the present. Your breathing is still relaxed and slow. You are still feeling relaxed, refreshed, and peaceful. When you wish to end this relaxation exercise, tell yourself that you can reach this gentle state of relaxation anytime you wish. When you open your eyes, you should feel refreshed, wide awake, and calm. Slowly open your eyes when you are ready. Remember, it is important to practice 20 to 35 minutes daily, in order to gradually experience a enjoyable state of relaxation.

☐ Case Examples

Both the progressive relaxation technique and visualization can be very useful for caregivers, regardless of the particulars of their situation. The following case examples describe the complex situations of three caregivers, and demonstrate how these techniques can be useful.

Ms. Brown

Ms. Brown is a middle-aged African American woman who has cared for her aunt who is in her eighties and has dementia. Ms. Brown's aunt moved into her home around the time of her eightieth birthday. It seemed silly for both of them to be living alone and, since they both enjoyed each other's company so much, it seemed like a natural step. At this point, Ms. Brown's aunt seemed very active and able bodied, but Ms. Brown had begun to notice that her aunt would not eat unless she was accompanied, her checkbook was unbalanced, and she constantly phoned Ms. Brown. Ms. Brown thought these problems would be taken care of once her aunt moved in with her.

And, it seemed easy for Ms. Brown to become the caregiver. She felt indebted to her aunt for the care she had given her as a child. Ms. Brown used to spend much time at her aunt's house when she was a child. Her aunt had no children of her own, so Ms. Brown was her aunt's "little girl." They had a warm, close relationship and Ms. Brown had many fond memories of all that her aunt had done for her. For Ms. Brown, becoming her aunt's caregiver was "just her": Her aunt required help and she merely was responding to a need.

However, the longer her aunt was with her, the more Ms. Brown realized how much assistance her aunt really required. Their relationship changed, and Ms. Brown started providing more and more care for her aunt. Providing assistance with personal care was especially difficult for Ms. Brown, as her aunt always had been so independent. The physical strain of changing dirtied undergarments, bathing her aunt, and helping her dress became overwhelming. Also, they seemed to have frequent conflicts, and they often would argue over how to do tasks and about how much supervision her aunt really needed. Between all of these strains, Ms. Brown found herself feeling more and more drained.

In addition to being her aunt's caregiver, Ms. Brown also worked full time as a director of a non-profit organization. She had a demanding job with long hours, many meetings, and regular out-of-town trips. It took all of her energy just to complete the tasks at work for which she was responsible. Between working and caregiving, Ms. Brown often was busy from first thing in the morning to late in the evening.

For Ms. Brown, progressive relaxation became an effective way to reduce her stress symptoms. Because she was going almost all hours of the day, she often found it difficult to relax. At first, Ms. Brown found it challenging to take the time to sit quietly and move slowly through the exercise; it was difficult for her to take her mind off of the many tasks she worried about daily. As soon as she sat down and was still, her thoughts turned to such worries as how she was going to rush home from work later to pick up her aunt from the local adult day care center, how she would manage to get her aunt to consent to a bath, and how she should use her aunt's money to ensure that she would get the best care possible. Also, Ms. Brown initially thought that she really was wasting too much time if she took 20 to 30 minutes for herself; she could accomplish many tasks in that time.

Gradually, Ms. Brown recognized that, in order for her to move through the progressive relaxation exercise, she would have to clear her mind and focus on relaxing each muscle. She started small by telling herself, when she had a distracting thought, that she could think about that concern later and should turn her attention to relaxing her body. And, once Ms. Brown began to feel the positive effects of being relaxed, she learned that the amount of time was worth it; she actually felt more energized to complete the tasks required of her. So, after trying out the technique several times and making an effort to take the time and concentration necessary, it seemed to work well.

Once Ms. Brown was able to recognize the usefulness of the technique, the next step was to determine when to use it and how often. Ms. Brown soon realized that doing relaxation techniques every morning before she started her busy day would help to reduce the amount of tension and stress she experienced throughout the day. By relaxing her mind and body at the start of every day, Ms. Brown found it easier to move through the day slowly, without trying to accomplish everything at once. Along with the relaxation techniques, Ms. Brown used visualization exercises to help her reach a place of quiet and serenity. In fact, she even tried out visualization at her church's prayer group that she attended two mornings a week and found it to work well. Ms. Brown liked to envision herself walking in the mountains around a cool, calm lake, with nothing to worry about. This served to be a point of focus for her while she was at work, trying to get everything completed before picking up her aunt. Because she took the time in the morning to visualize this peaceful place, she was able to reflect on it when feeling distressed and it helped her to relax during the busyness of the day.

Ms. Brown continued using the progressive relaxation techniques and visualization throughout her caregiving role. This was especially true during the period when Ms. Brown started facing the reality that she may have to place her aunt in a skilled nursing facility (SNF). She would pick up her aunt from the adult day care center after work, and then would spend the evening trying to bathe her aunt. Ms. Brown had to deal with her aunt's uncooperativeness and the physical demands of assisting with her personal care. Ms. Brown often felt exhausted after helping her aunt get into bed, but found it difficult to relax enough to sleep. She decided to try using the technique to sleep, and was successful. The same technique that helped her start her day and maintain a sense of control during the day also helped her go to sleep and get the rest that she needed. She experimented with different ways of using the exercise at night and found that listening to soothing music while lying in bed and moving through the technique was the most useful.

Once Ms. Brown placed her aunt in a nearby SNF, she found it particularly stressful to visit her aunt because she begged to go home. Even though

Ms. Brown felt she had the strong support of her church community, she found herself feeling exhausted and guilty when returning home after a visit. So, she tried using the technique to clear her mind immediately following a visit, and this also was useful. Although using progressive relaxation and visualization could not prevent Ms. Brown from being affected by the many stressors of caregiving, it helped her manage her symptoms of stress, and often helped her to better manage the challenges and tasks of the role.

Ms. Gomez

Ms. Gomez is a middle-aged woman who has been caregiving for her mother for several years. Ms. Gomez's mother lives with her in Ms. Gomez's apartment, along with Ms. Gomez's son who is in his mid-twenties. Her mother has dementia, and requires constant care and supervision.

Ms. Gomez has lived with her mother most of her life, from the time she was a child through her early adult years when she had a son as a single parent. In fact, Ms. Gomez's mother always has provided support for her: She helped out financially and with child care as Ms. Gomez struggled to rear her son in earlier years. Because of this, Ms. Gomez always has felt indebted to her mother. Several years before Ms. Gomez assumed the role of caregiver, her mother had moved to Florida to live with Ms. Gomez's sister and to be near to Ms. Gomez's son who was in Florida for a while and with whom her mother was very close. During this time, her mother began exhibiting symptoms of dementia and, because Ms. Gomez was concerned about the quality of care that her sister was providing to her mother, she made plans to move her mother back in with her when her son returned home.

The following years became much more than Ms. Gomez had anticipated. As her mother deteriorated and, due to the dementia, became more dependent, Ms. Gomez became increasingly frustrated with the constraints imposed on her because of caregiving. Her mother was very demanding and expected her to do everything. Almost suddenly, their once-close relationship seemed to disappear. Also, her mother increasingly favored her son, and demanded that Ms. Gomez do more and more for him. Ms. Gomez felt the need to be constantly available for her mother, and experienced unending pressure from her mother to also "wait on" her son.

In addition to feeling pulled at home, Ms. Gomez worked full time and had a lengthy commute to her workplace. Her caregiver role greatly affected her work performance, and she often found it difficult to concentrate and keep up with her workload. She was unable to be flexible at work, because unless she left the office promptly at the end of each day, she would not make it home in time to relieve the in-home worker who demanded to leave at a certain time. So, Ms. Gomez felt pressures both at work and at home and, as a result, easily became irritated and upset.

For Ms. Gomez, muscle tension was a part of daily life, and progressive relaxation seemed to help her deal with this symptom of stress. When Ms. Gomez first started using the technique, she was so relaxed by the end of the exercise that she began to fall asleep. It seemed as if she was so exhausted by the end of the day that, when she actually gave herself permission to stop and was quiet, she relaxed rather quickly. However, without the technique, it was difficult to set aside time for herself and her tension seemed to run from one day into the next.

In addition to using the exercise at the end of her day when Ms. Gomez felt fatigued, she also learned to use it to reduce specific tensions. Ms. Gomez found that, as she became accustomed to feeling relaxed, she also became cognizant of when she was experiencing tension and in what part of her body. She quickly realized that, when she had a conflict with her mother (particularly when it was related to Ms. Gomez's son), she would hold tension in her shoulders. Once aware, Ms. Gomez applied the progressive relaxation technique and was able to release the tension in this part of her body. Visualization added an extra measure and allowed Ms. Gomez to escape the stressors that surrounded her and to imagine a place that was calming. Again, she found this helpful following a stressful interaction with her mother, which seemed to occur daily. From this she gained a new energy. Ms. Gomez found the techniques quite helpful and reported that she continued to utilize them throughout her many years as a caregiver.

Ms. Schmidt

Ms. Schmidt is a woman in her forties who has been caring for her mother for several years. She had been living in St. Thomas and working at an art gallery, but returned to the United States after noticing her parents' need for care on one of her visits home. Her parents had immigrated from Germany when Ms. Schmidt was a young girl and, being an only child, she felt indebted to them for all that they had provided for her. After her father died, Ms. Schmidt moved in with her mother, and became her only and constant support.

Ms. Schmidt openly admits that she spent most of her adult life trying to "free herself" from her parents, and then ended up becoming dependent on them again. She worked hard to develop a healthy relationship with them while living away from them but, when she returned, all of her hard work seemed to dissipate. In order to care for them, she felt it necessary to give up all possibilities of working and to devote her entire energies to their needs. Their care needs were constant, and Ms. Schmidt thought it unacceptable to have anyone but herself fulfill these needs. After all, her parents expected this of her. Therefore, she no longer received her own paycheck, paid her own bills, lived in her own home, spent time alone, or nurtured her own friendships—all aspects of independence she had worked hard to develop. This, she says, was the most stressful part of being her mother's caregiver. Ms. Schmidt felt like she was socially, intellectually, emotionally, and economically putting her life on hold. She felt very isolated most of the time, and also felt hostile toward her mother because of all that she was sacrificing.

Ms. Schmidt was with her mother constantly, with little relief. Her routine began in the morning with waking her mother, dressing her, and transferring her to the couch in the living room. Then she prepared breakfast and tried to get her mother to eat. This was a challenge, as her mother frequently was agitated and uncooperative. After this was completed, Ms. Schmidt would try to get herself bathed and dressed, and then went about keeping her mother stimulated while at the same time managing the household tasks. She did not have a social life as her mother required constant supervision, and Ms. Schmidt found it challenging just to run out to get groceries and run errands. This day in and day out caregiving caused Ms. Schmidt to often battle feelings of anxiety and depression.

This was particularly true toward the end of her mother's life, when her physical care became increasingly taxing. Her mother was incontinent and pulled off her undergarments, often after Ms. Schmidt had bathed her. Also, her mother became "dead weight" and it was awkward to try to lift her out of bed, dress her, and sit her in the living room on the couch for the day. Her mother seemed to have more frequent mood swings and constantly was angry at Ms. Schmidt, making it difficult for her to have patience with her.

Ms. Schmidt often found herself tense and unable to relax; she constantly felt the need to think about what her mother needed and to be one step ahead of her. She agreed to try progressive relaxation training to attempt to mitigate this tension and stress, but initially was doubtful that it would work. First, her mother expected her to be at her beck and call, and Ms. Schmidt was unsure when she could set aside a time where she would not be distracted. Second, she did not think she actually could relax.

To begin, Ms. Schmidt tried setting aside time when her mother was napping in the afternoon, but she immediately found that she was easily distracted by the need to complete the tasks she usually was able to do during this time. So, Ms. Schmidt attempted to try the exercise once her mother was in bed. Although this allowed her to have time to herself, she found that it was not very beneficial because she never had trouble relaxing before bed, but did find herself feeling tense in the middle of the day. After some thought, Ms. Schmidt decided to complete the tasks that she usually did during her mother's afternoon nap in the evening after her mother was asleep, and to utilize progressive relaxation during the afternoon nap. This allowed Ms. Schmidt to experience the technique during the time of the day that she most needed it, and prevented her from being plagued with thoughts of tasks that needed to be done.

Once she had identified the optimum time, she then had to take the time to move through the exercise. It took several weeks before she was able to complete the entire exercise and feel the effects of it. In spite of her doubts about her ability to relax, she was determined to try to alleviate her tension. She started small and, at first, spent only 10 minutes moving through the relaxation technique. As she began to feel the positive effects of the exercise, she gradually increased her time to 30 minutes. Ms. Schmidt found visualization to be easier, as she immediately was taken back to the picturesque beaches of St. Thomas, which she had left several years before. This allowed her to return to a place that she had loved and to a time in her life that was more enjoyable.

After Ms. Schmidt realized that these techniques could have some positive effects, the challenge was to be consistent with the exercises and to continually make time for them. This was particularly true when she had a difficult day with her mother, although she quickly recognized that, on these difficult days, she benefited most from the techniques. With constant repetition and regular exploration of reasons why she was not using the exercises at particular times, she was able to integrate them into her daily life.

Over time, she found progressive relaxation and visualization to be effective tools in reducing her stress level. By using them in the middle of the day, she was able to go through the rest of the day without increasing her tension level. The methods became useful in reducing the sense of anxiousness that previously had plagued her, and they allowed her to continue caregiving until her mother's death.

☐ Summary

Progressive relaxation and visualization are interrelated, and they encompass a perspective on dealing with stress that caregivers may not have thought about much. They are methods that should be discussed with caregivers in-depth, to allow caregivers to fully understand them, experiment with them, and then use them on a daily basis. At first, caregivers may be reluctant to consider these ways of addressing stress, and the professional may be required to spend a good amount of time going over the concepts and practicing various techniques with them until they are able to realize their effectiveness. The end result, however, should be that caregivers have learned additional ways to deal with the stressors of caregiving. These ways may seem alternative to caregivers at first glance, but eventually may offer an innovative manner by which caregivers can approach coping with the daily effects of caregiving.

☐ References

Bernstein, D. A., & Borkovec, T. D. (1973). *Progressive relaxation training.* Champaign, IL: Research Press.

Carlson, C., & Hoyle R. (1993). Efficacy of abbreviated progressive muscle relaxation training: A quantitative review of behavioral medicine research. *Journal of Consulting and Clinical Psychology, 61,* 1059–1067.

Engle-Friedman, M., Hazlewood, L., Bootzin, R., & Tsao, C. (1992). An evaluation of behavioral treatments for insomnia in the older adult. *Journal of Clinical Psychology, 48,* 77–90.

Gustafson, R. (1992). Treating insomnia with a self-administered muscle relaxation training program: A follow-up. *Psychological Reports, 70,* 124–126.

Jacobson, E. (1929). *Progressive relaxation.* Chicago: University of Chicago Press.

Jacobson, E. (1957). *You must relax.* New York: McGraw-Hill.

Piercy, J., & Lohr, J. (1989). Progressive relaxation in the treatment of an elderly patient with insomnia. *Clinical Gerontologist, 8,* 3–11.

Scogin, F., Rickard, H., Keith, S., Wilson, J., & McElreath, L. (1992). Progressive and imaginal relaxation training for elderly persons with subjective anxiety. *Psychology and Aging, 3,* 219–424.

Woolfolk, R., & Richardson, F. (1979). *Stress, sanity and survival.* New York: Signet.

The Relaxing Events Schedule

The Relaxing Events Schedule is a method that can help caregivers gain control over their time; at the same time, it can allow them to experience a sense of enjoyment and gratification in the midst of the stress of everyday caregiving. The schedule can provide caregivers permission to engage in activities that are relaxing. This chapter will start by highlighting the issue of caregivers caring for themselves, and then it will describe the Pleasant Events Theory on which this strategy is based. The role of relaxing events in managing and relieving caregiver stress will be discussed, followed by an in-depth description of this strategy. To demonstrate how the Relaxing Events Schedule can be utilized with caregivers, the chapter will end with a case example.

☐ Caring for Self

Given the high level of burden and distress that caregivers may experience (Schulz, O'Brien, Bookwala, & Fleissner, 1995), one of the most elementary aspects of trying to help caregivers manage their stress involves caring for themselves. Caregivers usually will acknowledge that they must take better care of themselves, but rarely will do so. Most of the time, caregivers will take better care of their family members than themselves. They may routinely report stress-related symptoms, such as anxiety, depression, and fatigue. Also, caregivers often may experience feelings of anger, resentment, and guilt over not doing enough, even though they may spend 24 hours a day with the person being cared for (Zarit, Orr, & Zarit, 1985).

The burden of caring for a person who has dementia can be emotional as well as physical, and may lead caregivers to feel sad, discouraged, frustrated, or trapped; they also may feel tired and overwhelmed. Many times, caregivers put aside their own needs for rest, friends, and time alone in order to care for the person with dementia. It is not unusual for caregivers to feel alone as friends disappear, and they may not know any other people who are involved in caregiving. It also may become impossible for caregivers to get out of the house and they may become socially isolated.

Because of these typical factors, it is critical that caregivers schedule time into their routines to spend on themselves (Mace & Rabins, 1981). When caregivers no longer participate in activities that they enjoy, the greater is their feeling of distress and burden. It can become a vicious circle—the less caregivers do for themselves, the more stressed and burdened they feel; the more burdened they feel, the less they feel like caring for themselves. Caregivers can begin to feel trapped in a downward spiral. It is this very process that the Relaxing Events Schedule serves to address both by preventing and intervening in the spiral.

☐ Pleasant Events Theory

Lewinsohn, Munoz, Youngren, and Zeiss's social learning model of depression (1986) introduced the idea that pleasant events are linked to depression. Although people do not experience depression in the same way, depression typically is accompanied by feelings of hopelessness and helplessness. These feelings contribute to the attitude that there is very little control over life and the future. The approach of Lewinsohn et al. suggests that people can get help in controlling their own depression by working with a counselor who can offer encouragement and support while monitoring their progress.

In their concept of pleasant activities, Lewinsohn et al. asserted that, if one feels depressed, it is likely that he or she is not involved in many pleasant activities, or perhaps is involved in activities that do not produce much pleasure. When one experiences few activities that are considered to be pleasant, one feels depressed; when one feels depressed, one does not feel like doing the kinds of activities that are likely to be pleasurable or satisfying. It is similar to the chicken or the egg phenomenon: Does a low number of pleasant activities cause one to feel depressed, or does feeling depressed cause one to be inactive? Lewinsohn et al. proposed that it works both ways: Being involved in only a few pleasant activities causes one to feel depressed, and being depressed causes one to be inactive. This approach considers there to be a relationship between the number of pleasant activities and mood, and provides a potential handle on managing depression. By increasing pleasant activities, one can help oneself feel better. This model of depression, created in 1978, was used primarily with depressed younger individuals.

Although Lewinsohn et al.'s model was used primarily with depressed younger adults, a study performed by Gallagher and Thompson in 1982 examined Lewinsohn's earlier behavioral model as a way to treat depressed older adults. In their study, they evaluated three distinct forms of treatment: Lewinsohn et al.'s behavioral model, Beck's cognitive model (1967, 1974), and a more traditional brief relational and insight treatment approach. Participants in the cognitive and the behavioral treatment groups appeared to maintain gains longer than those in the relational and insight therapy condition. Those in the cognitive and the behavioral groups appeared to have acquired skills that they used on a regular basis over time. Skills taught in the behavioral model included overt and covert relaxation techniques, management of time, social skills, and problem solving. In addition, participants were taught to monitor their moods and track pleasant and unpleasant activities on a daily basis. Clearly then, this study raised the possibility that Lewinsohn et al.'s model could be applied to older adults experiencing depression.

Taking the application of the model one step further, a study performed in 1988 by Gallagher and Lovett demonstrated its use among the caregiver population. Given the reality that caregivers often find that time available for their own pleasant activities is minimized because of the constant, and often unpleasant, demands of the caregiver role, this study considered the link between caregivers' level of emotional distress and the number of pleasant and unpleasant events experienced. More specifically, they looked at caregivers' *self-efficacy* (individuals' perception of their ability to perform specific behaviors) for problem solving, using the model of D'Zurila (1986), and self-efficacy for maintaining pleasant events, using the model of Lewinsohn et al. They predicted that self-efficacy levels would be inversely related to emotional distress.

Results indicated several notable findings. First, in agreement with other similar studies, the caregivers in their study showed higher rates of depression than the general older adult population. Second, efficacy for maintaining pleasant activities and problem solving was positively related to caregivers' level of morale and negatively related to level of depression. Third, Lewinsohn et al.'s social learning model of depression, along with the social problem-solving model of D'Zurila and the notion of self-efficacy, appeared to be useful in approaching caregiver stress and the development of interventions. Last, the study suggested that psychoeducational classes are not always feasible interventions for depressed caregivers because they often are unable to leave their caregiving duties; more specialized interventions were recommended to treat this population.

It is interesting to note that the Pleasant Events Theory also has been applied with successful results to the care recipient population. Teri and Uomoto (1991) performed a study that assessed whether there was a significant relationship between depressed mood and pleasant activities among individuals with Alzheimer's disease, and also looked at the feasibility of training caregivers to be successful at increasing the level of pleasant events experienced by the care recipients and thereby improving their depressed mood. Caregivers were taught behavioral management skills to alleviate depression in the person receiving care. Although the sample was quite small, the results indicated that depressed mood was related to the frequency and duration of pleasant activities, with more frequent and longer duration of pleasant events significantly related to less depressed mood. Worth noting was the suggestion from the results of the study that caregivers who may be depressed prior to treatment also may benefit from the intervention.

☐ Caregiver Stress and Relaxing Events

Given the apparent relationship between pleasant events and mood among caregivers, there is reason to consider the application of this approach to caregivers experiencing distress. The fact that relaxation techniques can be used to relieve distress suggests that relaxing events is a more appropriate way to apply the Pleasant Events Theory to distressed caregivers. Similar to the Pleasant Events Theory, the Relaxing Events Theory holds that stress is a result of too few relaxing events and too many stressful events. The basis of the theory rests on the idea that the combination of the two produces and maintains the distress cycle and, in order to reduce feelings of distress and increase feelings of relaxation, caregivers have to schedule more relaxing events into their lives.

As a result of all the duties and responsibilities that caregivers must perform for their relatives with dementia (e.g., the seemingly endless demands on time, energy, money), it is likely that there are too few activities caregivers engage in that are strictly for their own relaxation. What is necessary to manage the stress is a balance between the nonrelaxing, but necessary, tasks of caregiving and the activities that caregivers find relaxing. By increasing relaxing events, caregivers can lessen their stress and gain some control over their distress cycle.

☐ The Relaxing Events Schedule

The Relaxing Events Schedule is a method to help caregivers take time for themselves. The technique requires that caregivers take time to identify events in their lives that they find relaxing and write them down in a calendar or a daily planner. The goal is to accomplish a modest increase in relaxing events. This may involve an increase in activities that caregivers have done and found relaxing in the past, or it may involve engaging in activities that they never have done before, but which they think may be relaxing.

The first step in helping caregivers develop a Relaxing Events Schedule is to have caregivers set aside a specific time to develop the plan in writing. According to Lewinsohn et al. (1986), this step is critical for five reasons. First, it allows caregivers to commit to the plan. The process of writing down specific events for each day of the forthcoming week formalizes an agreement and helps caregivers prioritize the relaxing activities. Second, planning helps caregivers find balance between the activities that must be accomplished and the activities that they really want to do. Third, having a clear plan permits caregivers to look ahead and examine if there will be any difficulties that may interfere with the plan. For example, if caregivers want to go to the movies on Friday afternoon, they may have to arrange for someone to come and stay with the care recipient. It is critical for caregivers to think ahead so that they can make necessary arrangements for care in order to follow through with the planned relaxing activity. Fourth, putting the plan in writing will contribute to caregivers' abilities to resist the countless demands that might otherwise conflict with the plan. Fifth, the process of planning will give caregivers a sense of control. Given the fact that caregivers may feel out of control on many levels, this is an important element that will add to caregivers' abilities to feel control over their time and, consequently, over their lives.

The process of setting aside time to plan the Relaxing Events Schedule often can seem overwhelming and almost an impossible task to caregivers. However, if the professional can keep these five aspects of planning in mind when discussing the schedule, caregivers will have a better chance of being successful. By making a commitment to write down relaxing events with activities caregivers really want to do, by looking ahead to make sure there are no conflicts, by following through on what is on the written page, and by resisting demands on this set aside time, caregivers will feel more in control and thus more likely to continue with the Relaxing Events Schedule as a tool to decrease their feelings of distress.

Once caregivers understand the importance of setting aside time to write down and schedule relaxing events, they are ready to start. The Relaxing

Events Schedule involves three steps. First, caregivers must identify relaxing events in their lives. Second, they must decide when to schedule events and write them in the appropriate space for the designated time. Third, caregivers have to follow the schedule.

Identifying Relaxing Events

In this first step, the professional should keep in mind that a relaxing event is a subjective one, since what may be relaxing to one caregiver may be stressful to another. For example, one caregiver may find going to a restaurant very stressful, while another caregiver may find this relaxing. It is important to allow caregivers to identify what they find relaxing, regardless of how it may seem to others. Caregivers may have difficulty identifying a relaxing event and it may take some coaching from the professional. Caregivers may have to think about years past in order to identify a relaxing event. It may be helpful for the professional to assist caregivers in identifying events by exploring how their lives were prior to being caregivers, what things they enjoyed doing then. It also may help to have them discuss activities that other people enjoy doing which they may wish to try; for example, they may be aware that a friend enjoys reading poetry and, although they never have done this, they may want to consider it. It is important to discuss specific examples of relaxing events; for example, talking with a friend, reading the newspaper, taking a bath, stretching and exercising, taking a walk, reading, watching a movie, or working on a hobby. Figure 5-1 can be used as a handout if caregivers are having a hard time thinking of a relaxing event. However, the examples should not be a substitute for caregivers' own lists, but should be used as a starting place to prompt caregivers to think of what they find relaxing.

The following case examples demonstrate the subjective nature of relaxing events and the fact that they should be simple activities. Ms. Rubinov, a 52-year-old woman originally from Russia, was caring for her mother who was incontinent and dirtied her clothes and bedding multiple times a day. This problem created an abundance of laundry that had to be done. When asked to identify a relaxing event, Ms. Rubinov explained that folding the sheets and clothes was very relaxing to her; she found the warmth and softness of the clothes a comfort. However, Mr. Morrison, a 62-year-old White caregiver, complained that, after working all day, coming home, preparing dinner, and helping his wife who was in the early stages of dementia get ready for bed, the last task he wanted to do was laundry. Just the thought of having to do it caused him a great deal of stress. Clearly then, it is important for caregivers to identify for themselves what they find relaxing.

Sitting in the sun.
Doing a project your own way.
Listening to music.
Going to a restaurant.
Exercising.
Watching a movie.
Talking about philosophy or religion.
Helping someone.
Doing a crossword puzzle.
Observing nature.
Planning trips or vacations.
Playing with a pet.
Reading a newspaper, magazine, or novel.
Learning something new.
Working on a hobby.
Laughing.
Taking time to relax.
Watching television.
Being with friends.
Breathing fresh air.
Eating a good meal or snack.
Showering or bathing.
Wearing informal clothes.
Having coffee, tea, and so forth with friends.
Thinking about your problems.
Singing.
Solving a problem.
Getting or giving a massage.
Having your hair or nails done.
Sleeping or napping.
Looking at the stars or moon.
Going to a support group.
Taking relaxation training.
Having peace and quiet.

FIGURE 5-1. Examples of relaxing events. Adapted from Lewinsohn's Pleasant Events Schedule, first published in MacPhillamy, D. J., and Lewinsohn, P. M. (1982). The pleasant events schedule: Reliability, validity, and scale intercorrelation. *Journal of Consulting and Clinical Psychology, 50,* 363–380. Used with permission.

TABLE 5-1. Daily planner

	Sunday	Monday	Tuesday	Wednesday	Thursday	Friday	Saturday
7:00							
8:00							
9:00							
10:00							
11:00							
12:00							
1:00							
2:00							
3:00							
4:00							
5:00							
6:00							
7:00							
8:00							
9:00							
10:00							

Often, caregivers may be hesitant to say that they have anything relaxing associated with their situation, and this usually is because they do not realize how simple a relaxing event can be. In fact, this was the case with Mr. Morrison. When he started exploring relaxing events, he identified many events that sounded very complicated to accomplish. For example, he thought of golfing, which involved arranging care for his wife, arranging for someone to play with, and setting up a tee time. He never considered the fact that sometimes just sitting and doing nothing was relaxing for him. It is important for caregivers to realize that relaxing events can be simple and they also should be realistic and easy to accomplish, so that the events themselves do not create additional stress.

Deciding When to Schedule

After helping caregivers identify relaxing events, the next step is to assist caregivers in taking the events that they have identified as relaxing and write them in on the Relaxing Events Schedule. Caregivers should be encouraged to write down at least one relaxing event each day for an entire week. Table 5-1 is a sample of a daily planner that can be used to schedule relaxing events.

It may be necessary to take a significant amount of time to help caregivers go through this process because it is likely at this stage that caregivers will indicate resistance to this scheduling notion. This resistance commonly takes two forms. First, although it is common for caregivers to acknowledge that they do not have many relaxing activities in their lives, they may be gripped by the picture that it is too overwhelming for them to think of *what* they can fit into their schedules. It is helpful to present the activity of scheduling as a chance for caregivers to begin changing this picture, and then suggest that the hour per week spent with the professional to go over the stress reduction program be the first item on the planner. For example, Mr. Morrison felt that he had no relaxing time anymore, much less time to himself. His first reaction to scheduling in relaxing events was that he could not schedule anything further into his week. It was suggested that the hour he spent with the professional going over Stress Reduction Techniques be the first scheduled relaxing event. Mr. Morrison agreed. Since he already was meeting with the professional once a week, this suggestion seemed like a good plan. Likewise, if caregivers already are engaging in some relaxing activities, these activities should be included in the planner so they are able to recognize what they already are doing.

In helping caregivers decide what events should be scheduled in, it is essential to reinforce that a relaxing event does not need to take a great deal of time and that it can be very simple in nature. For example, another caregiver, Ms. Hayworth, had listed reading the newspaper as a relaxing event but, when it came time to fill out the Relaxing Events Schedule, she questioned whether this in fact was a relaxing event since it usually took only 10 minutes. Once she was able to recognize that indeed this activity was a relaxing way for her to start the day and that, since becoming a caregiver, she never made time for it and instead found herself stacking the delivered newspaper day after day with regret that she had not had time to read it, she realized that it was a worthwhile event to schedule in. So, caregivers may require some reinforcement to help them appreciate the significance of scheduling in simple and time-limited activities.

Second, another common form of resistance is that caregivers may have difficulty recognizing *how* they can fit these events into their schedules; they may think that they do not have 1 minute to spare in the week to schedule in anything else. When under distress, it is typical for caregivers to generalize about their time. They may feel as if they always have to attend to their relative. For example, for Ms. Rolm, the most stressful aspect about caregiving was the fact that her life was controlled by the need for her mother to be supervised 24 hours a day, 7 days a week. She did not feel she had a moment to herself, let alone 15 minutes. For most caregivers, this is a common complaint. Often, caregivers will describe their situation as one in which they feel imprisoned. Ms. Rolm did not even think she could go to the bathroom without her mother calling her name or needing something. It is important for the professional to validate caregivers' feelings, but then gently challenge what may be a cognitive distortion, by helping caregivers break down how they spend their time. In the process of talking out her daily routine, Ms. Rolm indicated that her mother slept in until 8 a.m., and went to sleep consistently at 10 p.m. When the professional pointed out that this allowed some time in the morning and some before she went to bed, Ms. Rolm replied that it often was difficult for her to relax during this time for fear that her mother would awaken and need her assistance. After some discussion, however, Ms. Rolm was able to see that, by scheduling in several relaxing activities during this time, it would allow her to maximize time to herself and help her to relax. And, Ms. Rolm was able to recognize that her mother had never awakened during this time and that, although this was a very real fear, it was unlikely that it would happen. Even though Ms. Rolm was able to see her own cognitive distortion and, in doing so, felt less fearful of using this time for herself, she decided a further way to allay her fear would be to try out activities that would allow for interruptions by her mother. This example demonstrates the critical nature of the discussion between the professional and caregivers to help identify how to fit in relaxing events.

These two forms of resistance—the what and the how of scheduling relaxing events—are the most common, but certainly many more may emerge. During this step, caregivers should be encouraged to voice any resistance they may have about the Relaxing Events Schedule so that the professional can help provide validation, help them understand the resistance, and then move beyond it.

Following the Schedule

Once caregivers have identified relaxing events and decided when to schedule them in, caregivers should be encouraged to follow the schedule for 1 week. After this week, it is important for the professional to follow up and find out if the caregivers were able to complete the relaxing event as scheduled. If the caregivers were able to complete the schedule, a discussion should occur as to whether caregivers found the schedule helpful in terms of their stress levels. Reference to the Daily Stress Rating (DSR) Form will be useful at this stage to see if the relaxing events impacted caregivers' daily stress ratings. Typically, it takes more than 1 week for caregivers to see an impact on their distress levels but, at this early stage, it is helpful to allow caregivers to recognize the connection between the Relaxing Events Schedule and their stress levels. Once the association is clear, caregivers will be more likely to continue utilizing the schedule, with the understanding that it should eventually impact their stress levels.

If caregivers were unable to follow the schedule, the professional should investigate the reasons why, and help caregivers problem solve so that the following week will be successful. Some of the common reasons caregivers will give as to why they were unable to follow through with the schedule include busyness, an unexpected problem with the care recipient (i.e., medical difficulty, falling, not sleeping), tiredness, and thoughts such as "I'm not worth it" and "It won't help." Each of these reasons are worth exploring further, as they are often reality based. First, if caregivers found they were too busy to fit in the scheduled relaxing events, perhaps it is necessary to take a second look as to whether the events identified were simple enough and whether they were scheduled in at the best times. Second, if there was an unexpected problem with the care recipient, the professional should inquire if this consumed the caregivers' entire week or if it made it difficult for the caregivers to follow through. Often it is helpful for caregivers to realize that, if it did not take up the whole week, it could have been advantageous for them to go back to the schedule after the incidents in order to relieve the additional stress that was created. Third, if tiredness is given as a reason for not following the schedule, perhaps caregivers should try to complete the activities only 3 days out of the week. Assisting caregivers in taking small steps can help them take care of themselves; eventually they will be able to recognize that, even when they feel tired, the relaxing activities can be beneficial. Fourth, an in-depth conversation about the underlying feelings behind the thoughts caregivers may be having will help to get them to the next step of trying the technique. For example, after 1 week, Ms. Rolm admitted that she had thoughts such as "I'm not worth it." In discussion with the professional, it became apparent that, since caring for her mother, she had quit her job which was a strong source of self-esteem. Also, since childhood, her relationship with her mother had not been good, and she always had felt her mother was judgmental. Ms. Rolm believed that, since her mother had developed Alzheimer's disease, she seemed to be more critical and more demanding of her. Once she was able to talk about her thoughts of not being worthwhile and to gain awareness of the emotional source of these thoughts, she was able tell herself that indeed she had an identity beyond being her mother's daughter and caregiver, and that she was worth spending time on. Each reason given for lack of follow through on the schedule usually is reflective of the challenges of the particular caregiving situation and there is value in discussing each further.

Also, it is important to remember that setting a specific goal that is reasonable is a critical part of the plan. Caregivers should be reminded that it is more important to be successful than to try for a large increase in relaxing events, but fail to accomplish them. One way to help caregivers follow through with the schedule is to include in the plan a contract for rewarding themselves. Caregivers should include only those rewards which they can give themselves and that are not dependent on someone else's behavior. For example, caregivers may choose a reward of buying themselves flowers. This will help to reinforce how difficult the task is, but how important it is to their well-being.

☐ Case Example

The following case example demonstrates the role that the Relaxing Events Schedule can play in helping caregivers reduce their stress.

Ms. Sheffield

Ms. Sheffield, in her early fifties, has been caring for her husband who is in his sixties and has had Alzheimer's disease for several years. Currently, her husband is receiving care in an Alzheimer's care unit, but the years preceding his placement were very challenging for her. When Mr. Sheffield first began exhibiting symptoms of memory loss, Ms. Sheffield found it extremely stressful because it seemed that he purposely was being difficult. She often would get into arguments and tried intently to tell him what to do so that he would not keep making the same mistakes. This was one of the most frustrating periods for Ms. Sheffield.

Another troublesome aspect of dealing with her husband in the early stages of the disease was the fact that Ms. Sheffield was working full time. She had a good job in the defense industry, and had worked hard to get there. However, it increasingly became hard for her to juggle work and caregiving. Not only was it was difficult for Ms. Sheffield to leave her husband alone at home but, once she was at work, he called her constantly and it was almost impossible for her to concentrate on her job. And, when she was able to focus, she had a constant underlying sense of worry about what could go wrong at home. Likewise, once she got home, she felt tired from working and had little energy or patience to deal with the taxing aspects of the disease.

Once Mr. Sheffield was diagnosed, Ms. Sheffield was given educational materials on the disease which helped her to realize that the disease was causing her husband's behaviors and that he was not intentionally trying to antagonize her. Along with this understanding came the realization that he would continue to need more and more care. Mr. Sheffield was diagnosed in March and, in July, Ms. Sheffield made the painful decision to leave her job. Part of what made it so difficult was the fact that she knew she could never go back to the same industry because, during this time period, the defense industry was being downsized. So, Ms. Sheffield chose to give up her career because she knew her husband desperately needed her to provide him with 100% of her attention.

It was quite a change for Ms. Sheffield to be at home every day and to be solely focused on the care of her husband. Gradually, her role began to shift and she took on more of what he used to do. This shift was quite a stark one, since Mr. Sheffield previously had made all of the decisions in the household. At first, Ms. Sheffield talked to her husband about decisions but, eventually, she became the sole decision maker. Ms. Sheffield thought that she would never be able to keep up all that she was doing, as it seemed so painful.

An additional stressor in the situation was the reality that Mr. Sheffield had little patience, had a quick temper, and was easily agitated. Ms. Sheffield struggled to figure out how best to handle him. This was a complete change from how she had related to her husband prior to the onset of the disease, and it was a constant source of strife. She would argue with him constantly, which only seemed to upset him more. Slowly, she learned that arguing did not accomplish much, but it was a arduous process to learn a new way of relating to him that did not involve engaging his behaviors.

Although Ms. Sheffield had a lot of emotional support from her children, her son was a student at Stanford Law School and her daughter was a freshman at the University of California, Los Angeles, so their availability was limited. Ms. Sheffield was determined to care for her husband at home for as long as possible but she was afraid that, without much direct support, this would not be possible unless she learned how to manage the stress involved. It was in this context that Ms. Sheffield began learning the Stress Reduction Technique and, in particular, the Relaxing Events Schedule.

When the schedule was first described to Ms. Sheffield, she thought the concept was good and made sense, but she voiced great doubt that it would work for her. It was clear that she did not need to be sold on the idea itself, but that she would need a lot of assistance in applying it to her situation. Because she was able to recognize that since she started caring for her husband, she had stopped doing anything relaxing or enjoyable, she was willing to try the Relaxing Events Schedule and easily agreed to set aside time to write out the plan.

In approaching the first step of identifying relaxing events, Ms. Sheffield had difficulty thinking of what she found relaxing. It was clear that it had been a while since she had had time to herself for enjoyment, so it was necessary to have her reflect on years past to discover what she found relaxing. At first, everything she identified and described involved events that she had shared with her husband, and it was important for her to talk about her sadness of losing his companionship. It became evident that

Ms. Sheffield had done very little by herself and, therefore, it was necessary to reconstruct those events she previously had enjoyed with her husband into activities that she could visualize enjoying on her own. Also, most of the activities were complicated and would have involved a lot of coordination, such as going out to breakfast, going to a movie, or going to the beach for a weekend. While these activities were important ones for Ms. Sheffield to think about doing on an occasional basis, she was encouraged to think about activities that did not take a lot of time and could be done on a daily basis with little effort. After a lot of discussion, she identified several simple activities that she thought she would find relaxing: taking a hot bath, reading the newspaper, reading a novel, riding her exercise bike, and going for a walk.

The next step of scheduling these activities was an involved process. Ms. Sheffield was able to identify when she had time to herself, such as when her husband took a nap or when he was content to watch television. But, she was quick to add that these times were unpredictable and, when they did occur, she completed household tasks which were impossible to do when her husband was following her around. She was encouraged to think about whether there were any predictable times when she knew she had time to herself. This entailed a process of reviewing her typical week. After retracing the events of each day, she was able to see that her husband usually would fall asleep before she did, and she often would have around 15 minutes before she would feel ready to go to sleep herself. Ms. Sheffield decided that she would schedule in certain activities, such as taking a hot bath and reading the newspaper, at this time and that she would have a second level of activities she would keep in mind for those occasions when Mr. Sheffield took a nap or watched television. During those times, she thought she would try to go for a walk in the yard and ride her exercise bike.

After the first week of trying to follow the schedule, Ms. Sheffield reported that it was very challenging. She often found that, once her husband was asleep, she was so exhausted from the day, and so worried about the next day, that she could not follow through with taking a hot bath or reading the newspaper. It then was suggested that she try relaxation exercises during this time for the next week, with the hope that this would get her used to relaxing at the end of the day so she could integrate in these enjoyable activities. Also, Ms. Sheffield found that, as she had thought, when her husband had taken a nap 1 day out of the week, she immediately began completing household tasks she had found difficult to finish earlier in the day. Again, Ms. Sheffield was encouraged to try to change this pattern, and she agreed to make another attempt. A discussion followed that helped Ms. Sheffield consider getting a housekeeper to help with household chores so that she would be able to spend time with enjoyable activities.

After the second and third weeks, Ms. Sheffield had made some progress and seemed convinced that it actually was possible for her to follow through with relaxing activities, provided she took little steps each week. She found that, after trying relaxation exercises a few nights, she was able to clear her mind and get into a pattern of using the last part of the day to enjoy herself, instead of worrying about the situation. The third week, she managed to take a hot bath 2 nights out of the week and found that, on those days, her stress level was reduced. Also, on one occasion when her husband had taken a nap, she spent time walking in her garden and found that this gave her time to think about the importance of her role.

Although it took Ms. Sheffield several months to integrate relaxing events into her daily routine, it was a useful strategy for her. It not only allowed her to reduce her stress and feel that she was spending time on herself, but it also assisted her in the process of adjusting to her new position in life as a spousal caregiver without the companionship of her husband. In effect, it helped her to create an ability to experience pleasure alone, in a way that she had not done before.

☐ Summary

The Relaxing Events Schedule is a strategy that can seem very basic at first glance but, nonetheless, it is a key aspect of helping caregivers reduce their stress levels. Once caregivers are able to identify relaxing events and give themselves permission to engage in the activities, this tool can be a great source of tension release. It also fits in well with the other strategies that caregivers learn as part of the Stress Reduction Technique because, once caregivers are comfortable with scheduling in relaxing activities, they can apply this same principle to scheduling in the various strategies.

☐ References

Beck, A. (1967). *Depression: Clinical, experimental, and theoretical aspects.* New York: Harper & Row.

Beck, A. (1974). The development of depression: A cognitive model. In R. Friedman & M. Katz (Eds.), *The psychology of depression* (pp. 3–24). Washington, DC: Winston.

D'Zurilla, T. (1986). *Problem-solving therapy.* New York: Springer.

Gallagher, D., & Lovett, S. (1988). Psychoeducational interventions for family caregivers: Preliminary efficacy data. *Behavior Therapy, 19,* 321–330.

Gallagher, D., & Thompson, L. (1982). Treatment of major depressive disorder in older adult outpatients with brief psychotherapies. *Psychotherapy: Theory, Research and Practice, 19,* 482–489.

Lewinsohn, P. (1974a). A behavioral approach to depression. In R. Friedman & M. Katz (Eds.), *The psychology of depression* (pp. 157–178). Washington, DC: Winston.

Lewinsohn, P. (1974b). Clinical and theoretical aspects of depression. In K. Calhoun, H. Adams, & K. Michell (Eds.), *Innovative Treatment Methods of Psychopathology* (pp. 63–120). New York: Wiley.

Lewinsohn, P., Munoz, R., Youngren, M., & Zeiss, A. (1986). *Control your depression* (Rev. ed.). New York: Fireside, Simon & Schuster.

Mace, N., & Rabins, P. (1981). *The 36-hour day*. Baltimore: Johns Hopkins Press.

Schulz, R., O'Brien, A., Bookwala, J., & Fleissner, K. (1995). Psychiatric and physical morbidity effects of dementia caregiving: Prevalence, correlates, and causes. *The Gerontologist, 35,* 771–791.

Teri, L., & Uomoto, J. (1991). Reducing excess disability in dementia patients: Training caregivers to manage patient depression. *Clinical Gerontologist, 10,* 49–63.

Zarit, S., Orr, N., & Zarit, J. (1985). *The hidden victims of Alzheimer's disease: Families under stress.* New York: New York University Press.

Stress-Neutral Thoughts

This chapter describes the last strategy of the Stress Reduction Technique: Stress-Neutral Thoughts. This strategy is based on the method of cognitive restructuring which is a basic component utilized in the cognitive-behavioral approach to therapy. A brief history of cognitive restructuring will be provided to set the context, followed by a description of the role of worried thoughts in the stress process experienced by caregivers. Next, the Thought Tracking Record (TTR) will be introduced. The course of reducing worried thoughts and increasing Stress-Neutral Thoughts will be discussed, and the chapter will end with several case examples.

☐ Cognitive Restructuring

Cognitive restructuring is a key method utilized in many therapies that fall broadly into the category of cognitive-behavioral approaches (Mahoney & Arnkoff, 1978). Simply put, cognitive restructuring rests on the premise that thoughts (or internal dialogue) impact emotion, and that negative or worried thoughts generally are related to emotional distress; therefore, the most effective way to relieve emotional distress is to "restructure" one's thoughts, or replace negative thoughts with positive thoughts. Typically, when cognitive restructuring is utilized, some form of self-monitoring of thoughts is practiced.

There have been many influences on the development of cognitive restructuring but, given the purpose of this chapter, only three will be highlighted: Beck, Ellis, and Meichenbaum. Beck began his work in the 1950s and, by the early 1960s, he outlined the fundamental principles of his approach, which he called "cognitive therapy," in a series of papers (Burns, 1980; Wright, Thase, Beck, & Ludgate, 1993). Beck's model continued to develop and was published in 1976 in the book, *Cognitive Therapy and the Emotional Disorders*. Beck's "cognitive therapy" asserted that individuals' internal thoughts are directly related to the emotions that they feel. Specifically, Beck believed that an individual may have "faulty" or self-defeating thoughts, and these types of thoughts are directly related to emotional distress. He asserted that, by changing these "erroneous beliefs, we can dampen down or alter excessive, inappropriate emotional reactions" (Beck, 1976, p. 214). The goal of Beck's cognitive therapy was to help relieve this emotional distress. The means of achieving this involved helping individuals to identify, observe, and monitor their own thoughts (Beck, Rush, Shaw, & Emery, 1979). By helping one to understand the relationship between affect and cognition, an individual is able to alter distorted thoughts and, thereby, impact psychological distress (Corey, 1986).

Around the same time that Beck developed his approach to cognitive restructuring, Ellis constructed what he called rational-emotive therapy (RET). Ellis claimed that emotional disturbances "are the result of 'attitudes' and 'sentiments'" (p. 46) which are related to irrational thoughts. To Ellis, maximizing rational thoughts and minimizing irrational thoughts was the key to overcoming emotional disturbance (Ellis, 1963). Three steps are essential to Ellis's approach. First, external events that precipitated the distressing emotion must be identified. Second, the specific thoughts and underlying beliefs that make up the internal response causing the negative emotion must be determined. And, third, these thoughts and beliefs must be replaced with rational ones (Meichenbaum, 1977; Rimm & Masters, 1974). Assumed in RET is that, once people recognize their irrational beliefs, they will then wish to change these beliefs to be rational (Corey, 1986). Both Beck and Ellis applied their respective versions of cognitive restructuring to successful treatment of many disorders, including depression and anxiety.

In the 1970s, Meichenbaum (1977) articulated a notion of cognitive restructuring as an element of what both he and Mahoney (1974) called cognitive-behavioral modification. Cognitive-behavioral modification, according to Meichenbaum and Mahoney, viewed cognitions as critical determinants of behavior; therefore, cognitive factors can enhance the effectiveness of behavior modification (Schwartz, 1982). Within this context, Meichenbaum viewed self-instructional training as key to cognitive restructuring (Mahoney & Arnkoff, 1978). Self-instructional training made "subjects aware of negative self-statements" (p. 61) and Meichenbaum put the focus on the learning of problem-solving and coping skills (1977). He proposed that distressed people are different from nondistressed people in their learned means of coping (Mahoney & Arnkoff, 1978).

Beck, Ellis, and Meichenbaum made use of slightly different means, but all pointed to the central goal of cognitive restructuring: bringing about more adaptive thought patterns (Mahoney & Arnkoff, 1978). Beck's techniques were meant to allow clients to discover for themselves that their thoughts were self-defeating, while Ellis's approach was more straightforward and confrontational in that he focused on the destruction of irrational beliefs. Meichenbaum's self-instructional method, on the other hand, emphasized the development of a constructive set of skills (Mahoney & Arnkoff, 1978).

In addition to Beck, Ellis, and Meichenbaum, a more recent promoter of cognitive restructuring is Burns, who popularized this approach in 1980 in his best-selling book, *Feeling Good: The New Mood Therapy*. In this book, Burns (a student of Beck) presented, in simple language, effective methods for identifying "cognitive distortions" (p. 180) and replacing them with "rational responses" (p. 218). Burns presented the basic premises of cognitive restructuring in a clear and easy-to-read manner and, as a result, many people have embraced this viewpoint on treating depression and general emotional distress.

While the concept of cognitive restructuring within its many forms has been widely recognized and utilized since its inception, this is not to say that it has been accepted without critique. Many have pointed to the fact that worried or negative thoughts are not as maladaptive as the approach suggests. Coyne and Gotlib (1983) asserted that Beck's model is incomplete in explaining depression. Their research reported that depressed persons do present themselves negatively, but less consistently than the literature suggests. They proposed that equal consideration should be given to a depressed person's relationship to the environment, when trying to understand verbalized negative thoughts. Mahoney (1974) critiqued Ellis's approach on two fronts. First, he questioned Ellis's assertion that the discovery of irrationality in self-statements automatically motivates adjustment. And, second, Mahoney challenged the thought that "all forms of subjective distress are unreasonable" (p. 184). He suggested that, while it is obviously irrational to be extremely upset, it is not necessarily logical to be entirely without distress. In other words, the goal of eliminating all distress or negative thoughts may be the wrong goal.

Beyond questioning the role of negative thoughts, others have proposed that the relationship between negative and positive thoughts and emotional distress is more complex than that put forth by cognitive restructuring. Schwartz has written extensively on the connection between the two types of thoughts. He questioned the simplistic view that negative thoughts should be eliminated and positive thoughts should be increased, and has instead suggested that "negative thoughts interfere with coping more than positive thoughts facilitate it" (Schwartz, 1986, p. 599). Schwartz and Garonomi (1989) developed the States of Mind (SOM) model which proposes an optimal balance between positive and negative cognition's. This model suggests that it is the balance between the two that influences dysfunction, not merely the presence of negative thoughts. Kendall and colleagues also have contributed to the notion that the balance between positive and negative thoughts is critical. Hollon and Kendall created an inventory to assess internal dialogue (1980), and Kendall and others consequently put forth the idea that it is important to reduce negative thinking rather than just increase positive thinking (Kendall, 1983; Kendall, Howard, & Hays,1989; Kendall & Korgeski,1979). This pattern was dubbed the "power of non-negative thinking" (Kendall, 1984, p. 69; Kendall & Hollon, 1981, p. 110).

In summary then, cognitive restructuring can take many forms, but it primarily is geared toward changing maladaptive thoughts in order to reduce distress. Given this, however, one should not assume that maladaptive thoughts are the only element that may influence distress. And, one also should keep in mind that this process of restructuring thoughts is a complex one—it actually is the balance between negative and positive thoughts that is important, and relieving negative thoughts is more critical than just increasing positive thoughts.

☐ Cognitive Restructuring: Caregivers and Older Adults

Several recent studies have evaluated the benefits of utilizing some form of cognitive restructuring, within the context of cognitive-behavioral strategies, to reduce symptoms of distress among caregivers of older relatives. DeVries and Gallagher-Thompson (1993) demonstrated that, among caregivers experiencing anger and frustration around caring for an older relative, cognitive and behavioral treatments can effectively help caregivers manage these feelings by producing positive mood and decreasing anger and tension. Likewise in 1994, Gallagher-Thompson and Steffen demonstrated the usefulness of cognitive-behavioral therapy (as well as brief psychodynamic therapy) in treating clinically depressed family caregivers. In particular, the cognitive-behavioral approach seemed to be the more beneficial treatment among long-term caregivers of 44 months or longer. This suggests that, as caregivers experience stressors over time, there are clear benefits from structured, skill-oriented interventions rather than forms of therapy that focus on the sense of loss that is being experienced.

Gendron, Poitras, Dastoor, and Perodeau (1996) found that an 8-week group intervention program with spousal caregivers demonstrated the "potential benefit of cognitive-behavioral interventions with caregivers and in particular to the usefulness of assertion training and cognitive-restructuring (p. 13). Several additional studies (Gallagher-Thompson, 1994; Gallagher-Thompson & Thompson, 1995; Kaplan & Gallagher-Thompson, 1995) have demonstrated the use of this approach with family caregivers.

Cognitive restructuring, as one of several cognitive-behavioral strategies, also has been effective as a means of treating various disorders among the general older adult population, to which older caregivers also are susceptible. Morin, Kowatch, Barry, and Walton (1993) used this approach to treat late-life insomnia, and it was found to be a successful means of treatment. In fact, among the participants in the study, sleep improvements appeared to be maintained well at follow up, indicating that the cognitive-behavioral treatment produced durable changes in the sleep patterns of these older individuals. Stanley, Beck, and Glassco (1996) found that cognitive-behavioral therapy (and supportive psychotherapy) was effective in treating older adults suffering from generalized anxiety disorder; the treatment was administered through a small group format. Several studies performed with older adults who were experiencing an episode of major depressive disorder indicated the efficacy of cognitive or behavioral therapies with this population (Gallagher & Thompson, 1982, 1983; Gallagher-Thompson, Hanley-Peterson, & Thompson, 1990; Thompson & Gallagher, 1984; Thompson, Gallagher, & Brekenridge, 1987). Teri, Curtis, Gallagher-Thompson, and Thompson (1994) summarized 20 outcome studies and concluded that cognitive-behavioral therapies are useful in treating late-life depression.

The various studies mentioned, as well as the history of the effectiveness of the cognitive approach, make evident the benefits that caregivers stand to gain from learning these techniques. Given that caregivers deal with an immense amount of distress, ranging from anxiety to anger and sleep disturbances to depression, cognitive restructuring can be an effective tool in helping them cope better with the daily challenges of the role.

In applying cognitive restructuring among other cognitive-behavioral strategies with the older adult population, certain modifications may be useful. Gallagher-Thompson and Thompson (1995) suggested three factors to keep in mind. First, the professional should be active during sessions and keep the older person focused on pertinent topics. Second, these strategies may progress at a slower pace if the older person has reduced visual or auditory acuity. And, third, if compensation for cognitive slowing or sensory deficits is required, it may be useful to present important information in several different sensory modalities. These recommendations should help to ensure the success of utilizing these techniques with the older population.

The aim of the Stress-Neutral Thoughts strategy is to draw from the most effectual element of cognitive restructuring—namely, that negative thoughts impact emotion—and apply it to the distress of caregivers. The way that cognitive restructuring is used in our strategy is by assisting caregivers to identify worried thoughts related to giving care, and then helping caregivers to replace these negative thoughts with what we call Stress-Neutral Thoughts. This process takes into account the findings cited earlier in the chapter on the relationship of negative to positive thoughts; it focuses on neutralizing the worried thoughts, as opposed to just identifying them, and then increasing positive thoughts. It considers what Kendall called "the power of non-negative thinking" (Kendall, 1984, p. 69; Kendall & Hollon, 1981, p. 110).

☐ Worried Thoughts

It is not uncommon for caregivers who are under constant distress to have worried thoughts that often make it difficult to envision anything constructive in a situation. Often, caregivers' reactions to a stressful event can be determined by the strength of these worried thoughts. Worried thoughts often become so automatic that caregivers may be unaware that they even are thinking them. These thoughts typically are extremely negative and detrimental to caregivers' feelings of self-worth, and thus can promote the cycle of distress. For example, when encountered with a troublesome situation, caregivers may reinforce their distress by thinking such thoughts as: "I am not doing enough," "I can't handle this," "I should have done it this way," "If I knew what I was doing, Mom wouldn't be getting worse." Although these types of thoughts may seem very natural and understandable given the caregiving situation, they actually can induce increased feelings of distress. Worrying is simply a process of repeating these types of stress-inducing thoughts. Eventually, caregivers think the worried thought automatically, and they begin to feel as if they cannot stop the thought from occurring. At this point, worrying can become a habit—a learned behavior that repeats itself at different times in different situations. If worrying is viewed as a habit, it is reasonable to expect that it can be replaced with a new learned behavior that is productive.

Replacing these worried thoughts with Stress-Neutral Thoughts can help to lessen the perpetuation of the distress, and may even serve to relieve feelings of distress. Stress-Neutral Thoughts are realistic thoughts that reduce the threat of a particular situation and, at the same time, increase caregivers' self-confidence in handling situations. Examples of Stress-Neutral Thoughts include: "I did everything I could," "Worrying won't help the situation," "I've handled this before," "I did what I felt was best at the time." These thoughts all are realistic, but optimistic thoughts, and therefore can elevate caregivers' levels of self-esteem. They are the type of thoughts that can reverse the cycle of distress at any point. The key is simply in recognizing the worried thoughts when they happen, and then replacing them with Stress-Neutral Thoughts.

☐ The Thought Tracking Record

The first step for caregivers in replacing worried thoughts with Stress-Neutral Thoughts, is recognizing worried thoughts when they occur. The thought tracking record (TTR) is a tool that can help caregivers identify specifically what thoughts they are having, when they are having them, and how they are being affected by them. Table 6-1 is a sample of the TTR form.

The first column is for writing down the event that precipitated the worried thought. In the second column, caregivers should write down specifically what the thought expresses. They should be encouraged to stop for a minute and examine what occurred as a result of their thought. Finally, in the third column, caregivers should write down a thought that is more realistic and stress neutral to use in the future. Table 6-2 is an example of how the TTR works.

Caregivers often are hesitant to substitute Stress-Neutral Thoughts for worried thoughts because they do not really believe them. Although caregivers may not believe them from the start—and this is acceptable—it is important to go through the process anyway. As the new thoughts are substituted on an ongoing basis, caregivers will be able to accept them and they will become a habit, replacing the worried thoughts.

The goal is that, as caregivers continue this process, they will notice some changes in the way that they deal with stressful situations. However, changing habits takes practice and work, so they should expect that there will be times when they may not see all the differences that they may like. It is important for caregivers to keep in mind that, as they continue to replace their worried thoughts with Stress-Neutral Thoughts, the worried thoughts will soon dissipate and confidence-building thoughts will replace

TABLE 6-1. Thought Tracking Record

Day _____	Date:	
Situation	Worried Thought	Stress-Reducing Thought
Actual event leading to unpleasant emotion	Write thought that preceded emotion	Write realistic response

TABLE 6-2. Thought Tracking Record (TTR)

Date: 12/5/97		
Situation	Worried Thought	Stress-Neutral Thought
The adult day care center calls; they are unable to provide transportation for your relative today.	"People are always doing this to me." Leads to: Feelings of frustration and self pity, problem-solving ability impaired, stress level increases.	"They have been good to us in the past." Leads to: Clearer thinking, ability to problem solve, less stress.

them. Changing caregivers' thought processes often is the start of reversing or avoiding the cycle of distress.

Once the TTR has been explained to caregivers and an example similar to Table 6-2 has been presented, the professional should work with caregivers to identify a situation that has occurred for them during the previous week, and proceed to fill in the chart. If it seems arduous for caregivers to think of a stressful situation and identify a worried thought associated with the event, the professional may want to identify a commonplace scenario that many caregivers are faced with in order to help facilitate the discussion. One such example is a situation where a friend or relative urges a caregiver to place their relative in a nursing home. Faced with this circumstance, the caregiver may have the following thought, "No one loves my relative and they don't care about how I'll feel if I place my relative there." In response to this worried thought, a Stress-Neutral Thought would be, "I know they mean well and, by suggesting that I put my relative in a home, my stress would be reduced." This example may prompt caregivers to think of a real situation and identify a worried thought, and the discussion can then proceed.

Caregivers should be encouraged to use the TTR at least once a day, provided an event occurs that causes distress. It should be suggested that caregivers fill out the chart as soon as they can following an event that leads to a distressing emotion. If they do not have the chart when the event occurs, caregivers should be instructed to simply jot down the event and emotion on any available piece of paper, and fill in the chart later. If caregivers have difficulty thinking of Stress-Neutral Thoughts on their own, they should leave this column blank and it can be worked on when they meet with the professional. Also, the professional should inquire whether caregivers anticipate any problems keeping the chart, and if they do, the professional should work with caregivers to find a comfortable way for them to do so.

☐ Reducing Worried Thoughts and Increasing Stress-Neutral Thoughts

Once caregivers are using the TTR and recognize the importance of identifying worried thoughts and replacing these thoughts, the next step is to help caregivers realize that working on thoughts is a good avenue for change. First, caregivers' thoughts are always with them; therefore, they can work on them anytime and anywhere. Second, caregivers' thoughts are under their control alone and, hence, so is the ability to change them. These two points identify the fact that thoughts are within caregivers' control, and actually are something caregivers can work on within themselves, even if the situations cannot be changed.

Several techniques may help caregivers learn how to better manage and decrease worried thoughts. First, caregivers can use self-talk. They can learn to recognize that they are having a worried thought by using the TTR and, once the thought has been identified, caregivers can learn to interrupt the worried thought. For example, as soon as caregivers have a worried thought, they can tell themselves either aloud or internally, "I am going to stop thinking about this now," and then think about something that is stress neutral. This is one of the simplest methods of managing worried thoughts. A second technique involves having caregivers yell the word, "Stop," as loudly as they can as soon as they have a worried thought. The automatic thought will be pushed aside for a few seconds and they can then substitute it with a Stress-Neutral Thought. After some practice aloud, caregivers should be able to do this mentally and get the same result. Third, caregivers can utilize a mild punishment for a worried thought. Although this approach may seem ridiculous to some caregivers, it actually may work for others. Each time caregivers notice themselves thinking a worried thought, they can snap a rubber band worn on their wrists. Then, they can think a Stress-Neutral Thought instead. If this is done consistently, they will begin to catch their worried thoughts as soon as they occur, and the frequency will begin to decrease.

Becoming familiar and comfortable with Stress-Neutral Thoughts also may be a learning process for caregivers. Several techniques are available to help caregivers identify Stress-Neutral Thoughts with which they can replace the worried thoughts. One technique designed to increase caregivers' use of more realistic thoughts is to put together a list of stress-reducing thoughts. They should be put on 3 × 5 index cards, one thought per card. It may be helpful for caregivers to use the TTR to write some realistic responses to the thoughts caregivers already have had. The next time caregivers find themselves having a worried thought, they either should have a card available, or they can imagine themselves turning over one of the cards, and then they should use this realistic response to replace the worried thought. A variation of using 3 × 5 cards, or in addition to using them, is the use of cues. Caregivers can use frequent behaviors as reminders that they should have a Stress-Neutral Thought. For example, caregivers can remind themselves to think a realistic thought each time they eat, brush their teeth, talk on the phone, read something, get in the car, and so forth.

By using one or two of these techniques, caregivers are stopping themselves when they are having a worried thought and, at the same time, are increasing the frequency of their realistic thoughts. Therefore, they also are augmenting the likelihood that these realistic thoughts will become a habit. Again, caregivers should understand that it is most important to concentrate on breaking the cycle of worried thoughts, and it is not necessary for them to believe the stress-reducing thoughts initially. As these realistic thoughts become a habit, they will begin to accept them more and more.

☐ Elements of Self-Change

It is critical for caregivers to be aware that self-change often is difficult, and the process of changing one's thought patterns can be a challenging process. Four elements of self-change identified by Lewinsohn, Munoz, Youngren, and Zeiss (1992) can provide caregivers with a framework for approaching self-change. The first element is self-reward. Caregivers should be encouraged to make a specific agreement to reward themselves for sticking to their stress reducing techniques, such as changing their thoughts. The rewards or reinforcers can range from self-praise to having a special treat, like a walk in the evening or taking a weekend trip. These rewards should be realistic, obtainable, and under the caregivers' control. The second element is step-by-step change. It is important that caregivers be instructed to notice small changes in their thinking. For example, if they replace one worried thought with a Stress-Neutral Thought per week, they are being successful at their self-change plans. They should not expect to change all stress-inducing thoughts at once, because this is not a realistic goal. The third element of self-change suggested by Lewinsohn is modeling. Caregivers should imagine how some nondistressed person they like might think and act. They should ask themselves what their model would do to reduce their worried thoughts, and how they would feel about increasing Stress-Neutral Thoughts. The last element of self-change is self-observation. Keeping records makes it easier for caregivers to pay attention to their self-change process. It also helps with self-reinforcement, as it gives caregivers a clear picture of how much they are changing and how much they should or should not reward themselves. These four aspects of self-change are important elements to be remembered as caregivers are attempting to integrate the changes required in the Stress-Neutral Thoughts strategy.

☐ Case Examples

The technique of Stress-Neutral Thoughts can be an effective tool for caregivers to learn and apply. Although it may take some time, along with assistance from the professional, for caregivers to begin to see the usefulness of the technique, it can provide caregivers with many benefits in reducing their stress levels. The following two case examples demonstrate how cognitive restructuring can be used in helping caregivers reduce their stress levels.

Ms. White

Ms. White is a middle-aged, married woman who is one of four children and has been the designated caregiver for her mother for the past 12 years. Ms. White's mother always had been a very dependent woman, even prior to her diagnosis of dementia. When her mother moved to Los Angeles after being widowed, Ms. White began helping her with locating a new home, transportation, and daily tasks. Ms. White always was the strong, take-charge member of the family, and she had difficulty tolerating her mother's dependent nature even at this stage.

Then, Ms. White's mother moved to northern California to be closer to Ms. White's brother and to give Ms. White a break from caregiving. Shortly after the move, Ms. White's mother began showing signs of forgetfulness and seemed to require increased care. Not only did she have memory problems, but she also developed allergies, bronchitis, and emphysema; she was hospitalized often, and Ms. White made frequent visits as she doubted her brother's ability to manage her mother's situation. Over time, it became clear to Ms. White that her mother was deteriorating rapidly and was needing more and more help.

Finally, following one of her mother's numerous hospitalizations, Ms. White moved her mother back to Los Angeles to the home that she shared with her husband. Before long this was the source of a bitter conflict between Ms. White and her husband. He refused to help in any way, and provided no support on any level. He constantly pressured Ms. White to discontinue the care that she was providing for her mother, and eventually demanded that she place her mother in a facility outside of the home. Once

Ms. White went through the painful process of placing her mother, she soon learned that this did not necessarily lighten her load. She found herself making daily telephone calls to her mother as well as frequent trips back and forth to the facility to provide reassurance. Ms. White found it taxing to juggle the constant demands of her mother with her marriage, her job, and her own health problems. She also found it very stressful to maintain her relationship with her brother in northern California, whom she blamed for not providing adequate care and causing her to assume full responsibility of her mother. In addition, she found the physical hands-on care of others arduous; the stress of caregiving was physically hard on Ms. White's rheumatoid arthritis.

Ms. White frequently found herself overwhelmed with the responsibilities involved in caregiving. When the concept of Stress-Neutral Thoughts was introduced to her, she initially was doubtful it could help her. Although it appeared in conversation that she had many thoughts of a worried nature, she had great difficulty when it came time for her to identify those thoughts. It was suggested that Ms. White start using the TTR and begin with a situation that seemed to be a daily source of distress for her: leaving the care facility after visiting her mother. As this situation was discussed, Ms. White revealed that, when she left, she often had the thought that she was abandoning her mother. This was identified as a worried thought that led to feelings of guilt and frustration. Once this step occurred, Ms. White was asked to identify a Stress-Neutral Thought that could replace this thought. Again, Ms. White had great trouble coming up with this sort of a thought. The suggestion was made that perhaps a Stress-Neutral Thought would be one such as, "It is difficult to leave my mother, but I know that the staff at the facility will take care of her needs." Once this suggestion was made, Ms. White was able to distinguish between a worried thought and a Stress-Neutral Thought, and she indicated that she was willing to try to use the technique.

The next step was for Ms. White to practice replacing this particular thought as suggested. Ms. White was encouraged to focus on this thought alone and that, as she was able to realize how this could be helpful, she could then work to identify and replace additional thoughts. Ms. White made a commitment to try to use the method of replacing her thought every time she had the worried thought about abandoning her mother. After a week, Ms. White reported that, although she was able to recognize when she was having the worried thought, she was unable to take it to the next step; she actually found it troublesome to get her mind off of the thought. For the next week, Ms. White was instructed to practice interrupting the thought by telling herself she would stop thinking the thought. Then, Ms. White decided to try the technique of writing the Stress-Neutral Thought on an index card, and have it available to her in the car as she drove home from her mother's care facility. After the second week, Ms. White reported that interrupting her worried thought, and using the index card to remind her to replace this thought with a Stress-Neutral Thought, was working.

However, although at this stage Ms. White was able to utilize the technique, she again doubted the fact that this process actually would help her because she did not really believe the stress-reducing thought. She constantly was unsure that the staff at the care facility could help her mother as much as she could. Ms. White was encouraged to proceed with identifying and replacing her worried thought, even though she felt she did not really believe the Stress-Neutral Thought. It was suggested that the more the Stress-Neutral Thought became a habit, she would begin to accept it. So, Ms. White agreed to proceed with the technique, even though she was unsure it would impact her stress level.

After several weeks of continued working on this one particular thought, Ms. White finally reported that she noticed a difference in the way she was feeling, and that it was easier for her to leave her mother's facility. One positive outgrowth was that Ms. White found it easier to concentrate on her own work and household tasks on returning home, and therefore felt she was thinking clearer and was less distressed.

Once Ms. White reached the point where she was able to recognize the benefits of the technique, she was ready to go back to the TTR and identify additional worried thoughts she was having. Again, she started by recalling situations that she found stressful, and then used that as a springboard to identify the worried thought that was associated with each situation. It was hard work for Ms. White to get to the stage where she was able to accept the Stress-Neutral Thought for each worried thought she had but, after several months, she became convinced that this was a useful way to reduce her stress. Ms. White remarked that, while she could not control her mother's dementia, the fact that her husband was not supportive, or her own declining health, she could control her own thoughts, her reactions to stressful situations, and her own stress level. She also was able to see how her natural tendency to problem solve fit in well with the structured steps involved in replacing her stressful thoughts. Although using the Stress-Neutral Thoughts strategy was not a "quick fix" approach to her stress, Ms. White found that, with some work, it became a tool that greatly helped the way she handled the stress associated with the care of her mother.

Ms. Martinez

Ms. Martinez, a woman in her sixties, has been caregiving for her husband for the past 4 years, during which time he was diagnosed with dementia. Ms. Martinez had imagined her early retirement years would be quite different from the way they turned out to be. Although she had prepared to spend these years in close relation with her husband, she had thought they would be traveling together—both active and healthy. She was raised with the strong value that her role as a wife meant that she should care for her husband, regardless of how great his needs became. Her parents were from Mexico and, at an early age, she realized that caregiving was an expected part of being a woman and a wife. This value is a big reason why Ms. Martinez moved into the role of caregiver during the time she and her husband had planned on retiring, without ever questioning what it involved.

The role, however, was not one that Ms. Martinez easily embraced. The stress created by all of the changes seemed to be more than she could handle. Initially, she thought her husband was malcontent on purpose and felt he was aware of the arguments he seemed to be starting. It was painful to think that he was intentionally fighting with her and causing unnecessary problems. She asked herself, What is happening to our marriage? She also found it stressful to be forced into taking over many tasks her spouse always had done. Ms. Martinez was used to her husband being "in charge." Suddenly, she was in charge of finances, household matters, and decisions, in addition to caring for him. She felt angry about this shift and hated taking over his role in their marriage. How could he do this to her? Often, guilt would inevitably set in from her feelings of anger. She loved him, and wondered why she felt so much anger toward him. The interplay of various emotions and the shift in roles made the seemingly simple task of caregiving so overwhelming that she often was immobilized.

Mr. Martinez's condition made it almost impossible for the couple to attend social events. It seemed too burdensome to try to juggle light conversation with friends, while constantly ensuring that Mr. Martinez's behaviors were not causing problems for others. It became tiresome to explain his condition to others. Her other choice was to leave him at home, but she was uncomfortable socializing alone. After all, she had shared life with him for many years. She felt more at ease taking her husband to family events, but this was not easy either. She essentially was dependent on her family to take over when she arrived, so that she could enjoy the event. Getting out of the house for enjoyment took more and more energy and, consequently, Ms. Martinez went out less and less.

Once Ms. Martinez understood more about dementia and why her husband was behaving the way he was, it became easier for her to adjust to the changes. However, over time, he began to require more than only supervision as he also declined physically. She increasingly found it toilsome to care for Mr. Martinez, day after day. She did hire in-home workers to relieve her for periods of time, but this was a financial strain and she could not afford a 24-hour worker, which is what her husband came to require. Also, due to Mr. Martinez's reluctance to relinquish control over his personal care needs, the in-home workers were not always able to be very helpful. Ms. Martinez often found herself having great difficulty handling her husband physically during bathing and, on occasion, he fell in the process. The progression of the dementia and the demands of constant caregiving seemed to drain Ms. Martinez to the point that she often wondered how long she could continue to cope with providing his care in their home.

It was during this difficult stage that the Stress-Neutral Thoughts strategy was introduced to Ms. Martinez. Ms. Martinez was eager to try anything, as she felt she was experiencing more and more distress on a daily basis. It was easy for her to think of a situation and a related thought that was full of worry. For Ms. Martinez, the situation involved the daily task of providing personal care to her husband. As it became increasingly difficult to provide this heavy hands-on care, she often found herself thinking that she may need to consider placing her husband in a skilled nursing facility (SNF); she then had the counteracting thought that she should be able to handle the situation and do more to care for him and keep him at home. This inevitably led her down the spiral of distress, as she then thought she had no choice but to continue trying harder even though she was getting to the point of exhaustion in the process. Ms. Martinez was aware that this was a worried and unrealistic thought, but was not sure how to deal with it.

Although Ms. Martinez was enthusiastic about getting started in learning to use the Stress-Neutral Thoughts strategy, once she took the initial step of identifying the first worried thought to focus on, she was unable to move to the next step of thinking of a Stress-Neutral Thought. After much discussion Ms. Martinez was able to formulate a more realistic thought; namely, that she was doing everything she could to keep her husband at home. Once she was able to verbalize this Stress-Neutral Thought, she was able to say what before may have been impossible for her to say: that it may be best for both herself and her husband if she considered placement at some point. So, Ms. Martinez was determined, at this point, to begin the process of actually trying to utilize the technique by working on this one thought.

In spite of Ms. Martinez's determination, however, she reluctantly admitted at the end of the first week that she was unable to actually utilize the technique. She had been so busy with trying to cope with the daily challenges of caring for her husband that she had little energy to even think about focusing on her thoughts. Ms. Martinez realized that she needed something to remind her on a daily basis to identify when she was having this particular worried thought. She decided to utilize the technique of wearing a rubber band and write on it a phrase that would serve as a reminder. The following week, this method proved to be effective, and Ms. Martinez was able to identify the many times per day she had the worried thought that she should be able to handle the situation better than she was.

Once this identification was made, Ms. Martinez knew she had to move forward and actually try to stop the thought, and then replace it with the more realistic thought she had previously identified. She utilized the process of saying "Stop" out loud to herself when she recognized the worried thought, and this proved to be effective. Replacing the thought was a little more challenging because Ms. Martinez found it problematic to think a thought that she really did not believe. The values of her childhood seeped into her thought process and this new thought seemed counterintuitive. It took Ms. Martinez several weeks to determine that this was a worthwhile task, and she did decide to at least try to replace her thought. It did not come easily but, after 3 to 4 weeks, she found herself replacing the worried thought with ease and actually began to believe it.

This process was timely for Ms. Martinez as, during the same time, she was dealing with the painful decision of whether to place her husband in a SNF or to continue trying to care for him at home. Through this technique of replacing her unrealistic thought with a stress-neutral one, she was able to reach the conclusion that the best decision was to move forward in placing Mr. Martinez in a facility down the street from her home. The decision still was very agonizing, but she was able to recognize that it was okay for her to reach a point where she was unable to continue providing care for her husband at home.

Once Ms. Martinez placed her husband, she proceeded to use the technique in dealing with the many worried thoughts that resulted from the transition. Over time, the process became easier to use and she was able to replace her worried thoughts with less effort. For Ms. Martinez, utilizing Stress-Neutral Thoughts became a beneficial method of managing her distress level. It was effective throughout the entire course of caring for her husband at home, placing him in a facility, and learning to move on with her life.

☐ Summary

The Stress-Neutral Thoughts strategy can be a remarkable tool for caregivers to learn to utilize in managing distress. It is not necessarily an easy technique for caregivers to learn, and it may necessitate persistent instruction from the professional involved. Creativity in adapting the basic method to a particular situation is essential in helping caregivers embrace the concept. Caregivers may be tempted at various stages to give up the technique, and the role of the professional is to continuously reinforce the benefits of pushing through this stage to realize the full potential of the approach. After some time, and with ongoing support, caregivers should realize the usefulness of the technique and be able to adapt it to many different situations.

☐ References

Beck, A. (1976). *Cognitive therapy and the emotional disorders*. New York: International Universities Press.

Beck, A., Rush, A., Shaw, B., & Emery, G. (1979). *Cognitive therapy of depression*. New York: The Guildford Press.

Burns, D. (1980). *Feeling good: The new mood therapy*. New York: Signet Books.

Corey, G. (1986). *Theory and practice of counseling and psychotherapy*. Pacific Grove, CA: Brooks/ Cole.

Coyne, J., & Gotlib, I. (1983). The role of cognition in depression: A critical appraisal. *Psychological Bulletin, 94*, 473–505.

DeVries, H., & Gallagher-Thompson, D. (1993). Cognitive/behavioral therapy and the angry caregiver. *Clinical Gerontologist, 13*, 53–56.

Ellis, A. (1963). *Reason and emotion in psychotherapy*. New York: Lyle Stuart.

Gallagher, D., & Thompson, L. (1982). Treatment of major depressive disorder in older adult outpatients with brief psychotherapies. *Psychotherapy: Therapy, Research, and Practice, 19*, 482–490.

Gallagher, D., & Thompson, L. (1983). Effectiveness of psychotherapy for both endogenous and nonendogenous depression in older adult outpatients. *Journal of Gerontology, 38*, 707–712.

Gallagher-Thompson, D. (1994). Clinical intervention strategies for distressed family caregivers: Rationale and development of psychoeducational approaches. In E. Light, G. Niederehe, & B. Lebowitz (Eds.), *Stress effects on family caregivers of Alzheimer's patients* (pp. 260–277). New York: Springer.

Gallagher-Thompson, D., Hanley-Peterson, P., & Thompson, L. (1990). Maintenance of gains versus relapse following brief psychotherapy for depression. *Journal of Consulting and Clinical Psychology, 58*, 371–374.

Gallagher-Thompson, D., & Steffen, A. (1993). Comparative effects of cognitive-behavioral and brief psychodynamic psychotherapies for depressed family caregivers. *Journal of Consulting and Clinical Psychology, 62*, 543–549.

Gallagher-Thompson, D., & Thompson, L. (1995). Psychotherapy with older adults in theory and practice. In B. Bonger & L. Beutler (Eds.), *Comprehensive textbook of psychotherapy* (pp. 357–359). New York: Oxford University Press.

Gendron, C., Poitras, L., Dastoor, D., & Perodeau, G. (1996). Cognitive-behavioral group intervention for spousal caregivers: Findings and clinical considerations. *Clinical Gerontologist, 17*, 3–19.

Hollon, S., & Kendall, P. (1980). Cognitive self-statements in depression: Development of an automatic thoughts questionnaire. *Cognitive Therapy and Research, 4*, 383–395.

Kaplan, C., & Gallagher-Thompson, D. (1995). The treatment of clinical depression in caregivers of spouses with dementia. *Journal of Cognitive Psychotherapy: An International Quarterly, 9*, 35–44.

Kendall, P. (1983). Methodology and cognitive-behavioral assessment. *Behavioural Psychotherapy, 11*, 285–301.

Kendall, P. (1984). Behavior assessment and methodology. *Annual Review of Behavior Therapy: Theory & Practice, 10*, 47–86.

Kendall, P., & Hollon, S. (1981). Assessing self-referent speech: Methods in the measurement of self-statements. In P. Kendall & S. Hollon (Eds.), *Assessment strategies for cognitive-behavioral interventions* (pp. 85–118). New York: Academic Press.

Kendall, P., Howard, B., & Hays, R. (1989). Self referent speech and psychopathology: The balance of positive and negative thinking. *Cognitive Therapy and Research, 13*, 583–598.

Kendall, P., & Korgeski, G. (1979). Assessment and cognitive-behavioral interventions. *Cognitive Therapy and Research, 3*, 1–21.

Lewinsohn, P., Munoz, R., Youngren, M., & Zeiss, A. (1992). *Control Your Depression.* New York: Fireside Simon & Schuster.

Mahoney, M. (1974). *Cognition and behavior modification.* Cambridge, MA: Ballinger.

Mahoney, M., & Arnkoff, D. (1978). Cognitive and self-control therapies. In S. L. Garfield & A. Bergin (Eds.), *Handbook of psychotherapy and behavior change: An empirical analysis* (2nd ed.), (pp. 689–722). New York: Wiley and Sons.

Meichenbaum, D. (1977). *Cognitive-behavior modification: An integrative approach.* New York: Plenum Press.

Morin, C., Kowatch, R., Barry, T., & Walton, E. (1993). Cognitive-behavior therapy for late-life insomnia. *Journal of Consulting and Clinical Psychology, 61*, 137–146.

Rimm, D., & Masters, J. (1974). *Behavior therapy: Techniques and empirical findings.* New York: Academic Press.

Schwartz, R. (1982). Cognitive-behavior modification: A conceptual review. *Clinical Psychology Review, 2*, 267–293.

Schwartz, R. (1986). The internal dialogue: On the asymmetry between positive and negative coping thoughts. *Cognitive Therapy and Research, 10*, 591–605.

Schwartz, R., & Garamoni, G. (1989). Cognitive balance and psychopathology: Evaluation or an information processing model of positive and negative states of mind. *Clinical Psychology Review, 9*, 271–294.

Stanley, M., Beck, G., & Glassco, J. (1996). Treatment of generalized anxiety in older adults: A preliminary comparison of cognitive-behavioral and supportive approaches. *Behavior Therapy, 27*, 565–581.

Teri, L., Curtis, J., Gallagher-Thompson, D., & Thompson, L. (1994). Cognitive-behavioral therapy with depressed older adults. In L. Schneider, C. Reynolds, B. Lebowitz, & A. Friedhoff (Eds.), *Diagnosis and treatment of depression in late life: Results of the NIH consensus development conference* (pp. 279–291). Washington, DC: American Psychiatric Press.

Thompson, L., & Gallagher, D. (1984). Efficacy of psychotherapy in the treatment of late-life depression. *Advances in Behavior Research and Therapy, 6*, 127–139.

Thompson, L., Gallagher, D., & Breckenridge, J. (1987). Comparative effectiveness of psychotherapies for depressed elders. *Journal of Consulting and Clinical Psychology, 55*, 385–390.

Wright, J., Thase, M., Beck, A., & Ludgate, J. (1993). *Cognitive therapy with inpatients: Developing a cognitive milieu.* New York: The Guilford Press.

CHAPTER 7

The Effectiveness of the Stress Reduction Technique

When learning and preparing to implement the Stress Reduction Technique, an important question to consider is, What is its effectiveness? This chapter will address the question by first providing a brief review of the literature on interventions aimed at alleviating caregiver distress. While this review is by no means a comprehensive analysis, it will lay the groundwork for understanding how the technique fits into the larger context of interventions. Second, an examination of preliminary outcomes from a study performed by Bob Knight, Steven Lutzky, and Jodi Olshevski will provide a framework for understanding the effectiveness of the Stress Reduction Technique in reducing anxiety and distress, and how the technique compares to another method, the Problem-Solving Technique. Critical in trying to ascertain the usefulness of the Stress Reduction Technique are the qualitative experiences that caregivers have in learning and using the technique; these will be highlighted in the form of case studies.

☐ A Brief Review of the Interventions

From the emergence of studies on caregiver burden in the early 1980s to present-day literature, the interventions developed and tried in alleviating caregiver distress have been many, and they have differed in approach and method. Typically, interventions for caregivers have been psychoeducational

99

ure, teaching caregivers about the disease(s) affecting the care recipient and about common caregiving problems. Most have emphasized a mix
of group support and problem solving. See Tables 7-1 and 7-2 for a summary
of the studies that follow below.

Early reviews of evaluations of interventions with caregivers were not
encouraging. A review compiled by Gallagher (1985) looked at programs
that utilized education and support, behavioral and psychotherapeutic techniques, self-help groups, and respite care to alleviate caregiver distress.
She concluded that more controlled evaluations of the interventions were
needed in order to more accurately evaluate the impact of the intervention. Toseland and Rossiter (1989) performed a study that systematically
reviewed 29 studies on psychosocial group interventions which included
both education and support. Most of the groups were based on information
about the care receiver's situation, the group as a mutual support system,
the emotional impact of caregiving, self-care, problematic interpersonal relationships, the development and use of support systems outside the group,
and home care skills. It was concluded that impressionistic reports by caregivers and group leaders almost always were positive but, when structured
measures of emotional distress were used and when comparison group designs were employed, there was little evidence of change.

Several studies have tested different intervention approaches using im-
proved methodological designs. Lovett and Gallagher (1988) tested the efficacy of a 10-week psychoeducational program designed to teach specific skills for coping more effectively with caregiving. There were two approaches: The first focused on increasing the level of caregivers' pleasant
events and the second provided training in social problem-solving skills.
Both interventions decreased self-reported depression and increased self-
reported morale among the caregivers who participated. Greene and Monahan (1989) evaluated the effects of an 8-week group intervention with
caregivers that included group support, education about caregiving, and relaxation training. Results indicated statistically significant reductions in anxiety and depression among those caregivers screened for relatively high prior
stress levels. Toseland and Smith (1990) utilized an individual intervention
of 8 weekly sessions that included problem identification, problem solving, stress reduction, time management, and behavioral and cognitive coping strategies. Those caregivers who received the treatment demonstrated
significant change on self-reported psychological symptoms and emotional
well-being, as compared with participants in a no-treatment control condition.

While these three studies demonstrated improvement in design and results that are encouraging, they all either mixed dementia caregivers with
caregivers of physically frail older adults or used only caregivers of physically frail older adults. Therefore, it is unclear whether the positive out-

TABLE 7-1. Caregiver intervention studies

Author	Year	Intervention	Population	Type	Length	Measures	Outcome
Lovett & Gallagher	1988	Psychoeducational interventions	107 caregivers of frail older patients	Psychoeducational groups: life satisfaction skills, problem-solving skills.	10 weekly 2-hr sessions	Perceived Stress Scale, Philadelphia Geriatric Center Morale Scale, Beck Depression Inventory, Schedule for Affective Disorders and Schizophrenia (SADS), Index of Unpleasant Events, Reduction of Pleasant Events, Social Support Scale, Self-Efficacy Scale.	Both groups reported decreased depression and increased morale.
Greene & Monahan	1989	Support and education program	289 primary caregivers	3-component intervention: discussion, education, relaxation training.	8 weekly 2-hr sessions	SCL-90 Modified Burden Scale, Activities of Daily Living (ADL)/Instrumental Activities of Daily Living (IADL), cognitive dysfunction, psychological and psychobehavioral problems.	Significant reductions in anxiety and depression, little effect for burden and hostility.
Toseland & Smith	1990	Individual counseling	87 primary caregivers of frail older parents (daughters and daughters-in-law)	Professional counseling vs. peer counseling, problem identification, problem solving, stress reduction, time management, behavioral and cognitive coping strategies.	8 weekly 1-hr sessions	Bradburn Affect Balance Scale, Zarit Burden Interview, Brief Symptom Inventory, informal social support, Community Resources Scale, self-appraisal of change.	Participants receiving professional counseling demonstrated better outcomes on subjective well-being, psychiatric symptomatology, and perceived change in relationship.

TABLE 7-2. Caregiver intervention reviews

Author	Year	No. of studies reviewed	Types of studies reviewed	Categories of interventions	Results
Gallagher	1985	Not applicable	Not applicable	Education and support programs, behavioral and psychotherapeutic techniques, self-help groups, respite care.	Controlled experiments are needed to study the impact of various kinds of interventions.
Toseland & Rossiter	1989	29	Group interventions.	Support groups.	No clear link between participants' satisfaction and measurable outcomes. Studies with truly randomized designs have had mixed results.
Zarit	1990	4	Support groups and psychoeducational interventions.	Problem solving, respite care, support/stress management, individual and family counselors, support groups.	
Knight, Lutzky, & Macofsky-Urban	1993	20	Controlled studies (1980–1990) that attempted to change caregiver emotional distress.	Individual psychosocial, group psychosocial, respite care.	Individual psychosocial interventions and respite care show moderately strong effects. Group psychosocial interventions demonstrate small, but positive, effects.
Bourgeois, Schulz, & Burgio	1996	69	Exhaustive (15 yr)	Support groups, individual and family counseling, respite care, skills training, comprehensive, multicomponent interventions.	Support groups show evidence of improved knowledge, psychological gains, and development of informal networks, but only suggest quantitative treatment effects. Counseling provided for narrowly defined problems to individual caregivers is effective. Respite care appears to have only modest benefits. Skills training successfully changes caregiver behavior and, sometimes, patient behavior. Multicomponent interventions appear to contribute to positive outcomes.

comes would generalize to dementia caregivers. Also, two of the studies used quasi-experimental designs with nonrandom assignment to the no-treatment comparison group. In a more recent survey of the same types of interventions, Zarit (1991) noted that the few studies with truly randomized designs have had mixed results.

As is apparent, a difficulty in assessing effectiveness of interventions, by looking at both individual studies and reviews, is that the method-ologies used in the studies surveyed often are inconsistent. In attempt to correct this, Knight, Lutzky, and Macofsky-Urban (1993) reviewed arti-cles from 1980 to 1990 on psychosocial interventions and respite care for caregivers. The review was limited to controlled studies that attempted to change emotional distress in caregivers. Two criteria were used in select-ing studies to be reviewed. First, the studies measured caregiver distress, which was defined broadly to include subjective burden, depression, anx-iety, hostility, and other measures of negative affect. Second, the studies included a comparison group that did not receive the intervention. Meta-analytic techniques were applied to these studies. A total of 18 studies were examined, and no restriction was placed on the type of intervention used. Interventions included psychosocial approaches, respite care, and case planning.

This meta-analytic review concluded that individual psychosocial inter-ventions and respite care programs have had a moderately strong effect on caregiver distress. Group psychosocial interventions appear to have had a small, but positive, effect on caregiver distress. And, although studies on social and health care services other than respite care seem frequently to report important effects for caregivers, these effects do not consistently seem to include lowering caregiver dysphoria. A clear message sent by the authors is that interventions are most effective when they are targeted to caregivers with specific needs, and this targeting should be based on assessment of need and not self-selection by the caregivers.

In a shift away from examining outcomes and methodologies used, Bour-geois, Shulz, and Burgio (1996) reviewed 69 published manuscripts with a focus on the content and process of the actual interventions. They pro-vided a broad examination of both descriptive and quantitative studies, and grouped the studies into the following categories: support groups; individ-ual and family counseling; respite care; skills training; and comprehensive, multi-component interventions. Consistent with previous reviews, Bour-geois et al. found that studies on support groups demonstrated increased knowledge and psychological gains for participants, while quantitative treat-ment effects (i.e., perceived burden) were only suggestive. In terms of in-dividual and family counseling interventions, they reported that the liter-ature provides several studies that demonstrated effective treatment when counseling was delivered to individual caregivers. On the other hand, respite care intervention studies were reported to demonstrate only moderate benefits. The skills training intervention literature, which includes those interventions that change caregiver behavior and sometimes patient behavior, appear to provide the "most robust and rigorously evaluated treatments," according to Bourgeois et al. (p. 77). And, last, what the authors called multicomponent interventions (comprehensive service delivery programs) appeared to add to positive outcomes for caregivers who were interested in the program offerings.

Bourgeois et al. concluded that measurement validity is important, but should not disguise the importance of clinical impact. They suggested that it is not just statistical significance and consistent methodology that is important in looking at interventions, but whether caregivers actually feel that their involvement in the intervention helped to significantly alter their own or their families' lives. They proposed that the critical factors to ensure an intervention is effective are determination of caregivers' needs, expectations of the intervention, and realistic treatment goals.

The literature on caregiver interventions, then, offers several insights to evaluating the effectiveness of the Stress Reduction Technique. First, the success of the technique is dependent not just on the strategies themselves, but also on how the intervention is targeted, described, and applied to caregivers' situations. Second, in the context of the various interventions reviewed, the Stress Reduction Technique can be viewed in a number of ways, given the inconsistent terminology used in categorizing treatment studies. In terms of the meta-analytic study by Knight et al. (1993), the Stress Reduction Technique could be considered an "individual psychosocial intervention" (p. 246); while according to the review by Bourgeois et al. (1996), the Stress Reduction Technique could be considered either an "individual and family counseling" (pp. 72–73) intervention or a "skills training" (pp. 75–77) intervention. In either case, it is apparent that the type of intervention provided by the Stress Reduction Technique fits into categories that have shown fairly effective treatment results.

In order to gain a more precise picture of how the Stress Reduction Technique impacts caregiver distress, an examination will now be made of the preliminary outcomes from a study performed by Knight, Lutzky, and Olshevski.

☐ The Effects of Psychoeducational Intervention on Self-Reported Distress in Caregivers

The study involved an 8-week psychoeducational program of individual tutoring in stress reduction training as well as problem-solving training. Participants were randomly assigned either to the stress reduction training, the problem-solving training, or a wait list. All participants were primary caregivers of older adults with dementia and were prescreened for high levels of burden. Prescreening for high levels of perceived stress assured that caregivers needed the intervention and minimized the possibility of floor effects for change in outcome variables.

Stress reduction training emphasized the caregiver's own emotional state. Caregivers were taught to monitor distress levels on a daily basis, to use progressive relaxation, to plan relaxing activities on a weekly basis, and to change stress enhancing thoughts to stress reducing or Stress-Neutral Thoughts. The problem-solving training focused more on improving the caregiver's problem-solving ability and ability to manage the care recipient. This model followed the Zarit, Orr, and Zarit (1985) approach and focused on monitoring the care recipient's behavior, devising behavioral management strategies to solve the older adult's care problems, and evaluating and refining these interventions.

Method

Subjects

The participants were selected from a larger investigation of caregiver distress on the basis of high scores on the Zarit Burden Interview (ZBI; Zarit, Reever, & Bach-Peterson, 1980). The larger sample was recruited from caregivers of older adults with dementia who contacted the telephone information lines of the Alzheimer's Association of Los Angeles County or the Los Angeles Caregiver Resource Center (a social service program for caregivers of adults with brain impairments). All were caregivers of persons with a dementing illness, and either lived with the recipient or provided more than 8 hours per week of care. All caregivers in the larger sample who scored 40 or more on the ZBI were asked to participate in the intervention study. Seventy-four of 121 caregivers met this requirement. High burden caregivers were randomly assigned to stress reduction training, problem-solving training, or to the wait list. Persons assigned to the wait list were reinterviewed 8 weeks later, and then randomly assigned to one of the two intervention conditions. All subjects were interviewed within 2 weeks after the end of the intervention, and then again for a follow-up assessment approximately 2 months after the intervention ended. Fifty of the 74 caregivers completed the 8-week intervention or wait list period and the posttest assessment.

Measures

The screening variable used, as previously mentioned, was the ZBI. Several scales were used to measure caregivers' self-reported distress: the Brief

Symptom Inventory, the Spielberger State-Trait Anxiety Inventory, and the Center for Epidemiological Studies Depression Scale. Systolic blood pressure-reactivity (SBP-R) also was measured by an Orion biofeedback monitor with a SC 700A automatic blood pressure cuff. Systolic blood pressure was sampled once per 3-minute interval during each of three 12-minute periods with the mean of the four 3-minute samples used as the measure for each task (a rest period and two task periods). One stress task was a mental effort task (counting backward by 7s from 500). The other task was to discuss the most stressful caregiving problem that occurred in the preceding month. Cardiovascular reactivity (CVR) was calculated as the difference between mean systolic blood pressure for each task period minus the mean for the rest period. And, last, cognitive coping styles of caregivers were measured by the Folkman and Lazarus scale (1988).

Procedure

The initial interview consisted of demographic questions, questions about the circumstances of the caregiving situation, the paper-and-pencil self-report questionnaires, the CVR procedure, and the coping questionnaire. Interviews were conducted in the caregiver's home or on campus at the caregiver's convenience. Initial interviews averaged about 3 hours in length. The intervention sessions lasted about 1 hour each and were scheduled weekly for 8 weeks. After material was introduced, there was considerable emphasis on practicing techniques. Caregivers were encouraged to provide feedback on results and the trainers provided troubleshooting advice on how to use the techniques to optimum effect.

Design

The paper-and-pencil measures and the CVR procedure were given at the initial interview and were repeated within 2 weeks of the final treatment session (posttest). The test of initial outcomes compares the three groups at posttest using a doubly multivariate repeated measures ANOVA. With the crossover design, wait list subjects went into treatment after 8 weeks on the wait list and posttest, and then were retested after treatment (treatment posttest) and for the 2-month follow up. The test of maintenance of gain at follow up includes wait list subjects in the two treatment groups and compares stress reduction training to problem-solving training using a doubly multivariate repeated measures ANOVA of scores at pretest, treatment posttest, and follow up. In addition, correlational analyses were conducted to explore whether changes in process variables would predict changes in outcome measures.

Results

Outcome Measures

The three-group comparison of stress reduction training, problem-solving training, and wait list was analyzed with a doubly multivariate repeated measures MANOVA. Since the sample size for this analysis is small, the averaged univariate F test was used because it has greater power with small samples. The Maunchly sphericity test rejected the assumptions of equal variances and zero covariances in the covariance matrix (chi-square $= 218.8$, $p < .001$). The degrees of freedom for the repeated measures test were adjusted using the Huynh-Feldt epsilon correction. The treatment × time interaction effect was significant (F (7, 40) $= 2.61$, $p < .01$). Neither the main effect for treatment nor the main effect for time were significant. The associated univariate tests show that this effect is due to change in systolic reactivity during caregiving story, to change in Global Symptom Index (GSI), and to change in state anxiety. Tukey's post hoc comparisons of group means with alpha set at .05 reveal that these differences are due to stress reduction training being superior to wait list in reduction of state anxiety and in reduction of GSI. Stress reduction training was more effective than problem-solving training in reducing state anxiety. SBP-R *increased* significantly more in the problem-solving training as compared to stress reduction training. No comparisons of the problem-solving group and the wait list reached significance. However, the standard deviation of SBP-R was considerably higher in the wait list group than in the interventions; if the standard error was based on the pooled variance of the other groups, the SBP-R change in the problem-solving group would be significantly higher than the wait list group.

In assessing the follow-up effects, the Maunchly sphericity test again was significant (chi-square $= 329.0$, $p < .001$) and so the Huynh-Feldt epsilon was used to adjust degrees of freedom for the averaged F test. The main effect for time was significant (F (6,54) $= 2.33$, $p < .05$). The associated univariate tests suggest that this effect was due to change in GSI and in state anxiety. Planned post hoc paired t tests were performed using a Bonferroni correction. GSI and state anxiety showed significant change from baseline to immediate posttest (t (37) $= 3.63$ and 2.75 respectively, $p < .009$). Neither GSI nor state anxiety showed a significant difference between immediate posttest and 2-month follow up. The direct comparison of baseline to follow up shows that GSI is significantly different (t (30) $=$ 3.30, $p < .002$); however, state anxiety is not different from baseline at follow up, suggesting a tendency to rebound once treatment is terminated. Neither main effect for group nor the group by time interaction effects were significant. The group by time interaction approached significance; given the low power of this test, the failure to reach significance must be considered inconclusive.

Process Measures

Correlational analyses were used to see if changes in process variables predicted changes in outcome variables. In stress reduction training, declines in the use of escape avoidance strategies and in the use of distancing predicted lowered CVR ($r = .40$ and $.52$) respectively, ($p < .05$). Lower use of self-blame led to declines in GSI and state anxiety ($r = .45$ and $.52$) respectively, ($p < .05$). In the problem-solving training group, increased use of self-control strategies was associated with higher CVR ($r = .56$).

Discussion

Although the results of this randomized evaluation of psychoeducational interventions for dementia caregivers should be viewed as preliminary, they provide support for the effectiveness of using Stress Reduction Techniques with this population. Stress reduction training appears to have an effect on psychological symptoms and state anxiety at posttest and this effect does not change significantly over a 2-month follow up. In contrast, caregivers showed increased cardiovascular reactivity in the problem-solving condition. While further study with larger samples clearly is needed, the Stress Reduction Technique appears to be more effective than the problem-solving training in lowering anxiety.

The experimental outcome data and the correlational data on processes tend to confirm the premise of stress and coping models for understanding the distress of this population and for designing interventions to assist them. These findings strengthen the evidence for the effectiveness of psychological approaches to helping dementia caregivers by adding experimental evidence to the quasi-experimental designs of Greene and Monahan (1989) and Toseland and Smith (1990). Along with these earlier studies, this investigation supports the importance of prescreening caregivers for interventions, a step which arguably equates caregiver intervention studies with other intervention studies which use subjects that have a clinical diagnosis or who are actively seeking clinical treatment.

The correlations between changes in cognitive coping styles during psychoeducational interventions and change in SBP-R can begin to extend our understanding of the role of coping responses in changing psychophysiological stress responses. The study showed that decreased use of escapist coping is correlated with lower levels of CVR. The finding that less use of distancing was correlated with lower CVR in stress reduction training and that higher CVR levels in the problem-solving technique were correlated with increased use of self-control strategies, support the argument that suppression of emotions leads to increased psychophysiological distress (see Rodin & Salovey, 1989). These tentative findings on coping styles suggest that interventions should work on decreasing avoidant coping and self-blame and on increasing emotional expression. A lower frequency of self-blame (accepting responsibility) also led to less anxiety in the stress reduction training condition. The effects on CVR and the correlation of CVR to coping styles provides empirical support for the use of psychophysiological outcome measures and for links between coping styles and CVR.

There clearly are limitations in this investigation that need to be considered in generalizing the findings. The small size of the sample limits the power of the statistical tests and clearly calls for replication. The small sample also precludes testing for specific treatment effects by subgroups (gender, relationship to recipient, ethnicity). Also, the attrition over repeated times of testing affects the generalizability of the results in unknown ways.

☐ Case Examples

The preceding study points toward the effectiveness of the Stress Reduction Technique as evaluated by quantitative methods. Also important in assessing the effectiveness of the technique is looking at how an individual caregiver has experienced the technique and whether, on an individual level, a caregiver finds it helpful in reducing the level of distress. The following two cases demonstrate this point.

Ms. Groth

Ms. Groth has been a caregiver for her husband for over 3 years. She is a woman in her late fifties and her husband is many years older. Her husband not only has dementia but also is bedbound and requires almost total care, needing attention around the clock. According to Ms. Groth, her husband's care is somewhat easier now, compared to the time during which he was ambulatory and she felt as if she had to follow him around all the time to make sure he did not place himself in danger. However, although he no longer requires the vigilance of Ms. Groth in following him around, he cannot be left alone due to his extensive care needs. And, he requires heavy hands-on care, such as lifting, turning, changing incontinence undergarments, and bathing, all of which Ms. Groth finds physically exhausting.

Ms. Groth has been the primary caregiver for her husband. Although her daughter lives in a small house behind Ms. Groth's home, she has a husband and a young daughter and has not been available on a regular basis to relieve Ms. Groth of the tasks of helping her husband with personal care. Ms. Groth also has a son, but he does not live nearby and has been unable to assist much with the hands-on care.

Ms. Groth has found the role of caregiving to be very distressing. In fact, she has reported frequently feeling depressed. She has felt trapped by having to remain in her home almost constantly to ensure care for her husband's needs. She has hated the routine and the confinement. And, since her husband is so much older than herself, she has felt this role was placed on her prematurely. She is at the age where she wants to enjoy having her children grown and out of the house, and she has plenty of things that she had intended to do during this time in her life. She also has felt that she has been unable to enjoy her granddaughter as much as she wished. It has seemed as if the only time she has been able to spend with her has been when her granddaughter has come over to the house, and then Ms. Groth has been unable to enjoy her entirely because she always has been distracted by her husband's needs. Also, Ms. Groth has felt that her granddaughter has not been able to truly enjoy her as a grandmother; she speculates that her granddaughter has been resentful that her grandmother has had to tend to her sick grandfather instead of playing with her for hours.

Ms. Groth has had some formal support as a visiting nurse has stopped by on a weekly basis to check her husband's vitals, but this never has been long enough to relieve her of her responsibilities. It has only given her 15 minutes to run to the store and get groceries. Ms. Groth also has seemed reluctant to accept additional formal help. She has felt that she has the best sense of how to care for her husband since he often has been resistant to receiving care and she has had to coerce him into turning or getting bathed.

It was in this context that Ms. Groth started to learn the Stress Reduction Technique. Clearly, she had a high level of distress, both in terms of self-report and also as indicated by the screening tool. As the various methods were taught to Ms. Groth, she seemed very eager to learn them. When she talked about her caregiving situation and what was most difficult, she often was tearful and angry. Although she was ready for any and all help available, the most challenging aspect of utilizing the technique was trying to find the time required, and trying to do this on a consistent basis.

Often this would be so frustrating to her that, during weekly sessions, it seemed necessary to let her talk about her frustrations first, and then gently try to help her identify ways that she could try using the methods. For example, she found it impossible to find 20 minutes a day when she could be alone and not interrupted by her husband's cries for help. She wanted to try using relaxation techniques, but just could not seem to do it. Discussion about her time revealed that her husband did seem to sleep for 6 hours at night, and this often was the time when she tried to get household tasks done before sleeping herself for around 5 hours per night. After some ideas were brought up about how she could take care of the household tasks in other ways, it was suggested that she try utilizing the relaxation technique once her husband was asleep and she was ready to go to sleep. After a week of trying this, Ms. Groth reported that she was able to use relaxation two times during the week, and that it helped her to feel rested, relaxed, and ready to face the next day. It was this type of problem solving that was necessary to help Ms. Groth actually use the various Stress Reduction Techniques. At the end of the sessions, she seemed to have identified ways to make the time necessary for her to use the methods she had been taught. Ms. Groth also reported that she felt better about her ability to manage her feelings of stress but, clearly, her caregiver role would continue to cause distress and only time would reveal how effective the technique would be for her.

A follow-up interview was arranged with Ms. Groth approximately 2 years after she had received the training sessions on the Stress Reduction Technique. Her husband had continued to deteriorate, had become nonverbal, and required a feeding tube. Although she reported that his worsening condition was difficult, she also had the sense that he was at the latter stages of his life and this gave her hope that the end was imminent. At the same time, she reported feeling afraid of the end of her role, since she had grown accustomed to it. She indicated that she had a sense of satisfaction about caregiving in that she was doing something good. Ms. Groth also voiced a strong sense that she was better off as a person as a result of caregiving, and that she had moved beyond her anger into understanding and acceptance of the situation. She felt as if she had become a stronger person, both mentally and physically.

The formal supports Ms. Groth utilized had increased. She had a visiting nurse two times per week; a home health aide for bathing three times per week; and an aide 4 hours per day, 4 days per week for a period of time. Also, her son had moved in with her, and he helped with care at night and with lifting. Ms. Groth also had accessed her neighbors and friends for emotional support.

In reflecting on the Stress Reduction Technique and whether it was helpful, Ms. Groth reported that she clearly had benefited from it and that it had helped her immensely. She had found it useful to think about replacing her worried thoughts and had written out Stress-Neutral Thoughts on cards which she used frequently. She continued to use relaxation and visualization at night, and found this very beneficial. Ms. Groth also was now in the habit of spending an hour per day on herself, which had grown out of the technique of identifying and scheduling relaxing events. She said this was especially helpful to her.

So, Ms. Groth is an example of a caregiver who seemed to benefit greatly from the Stress Reduction Technique and, for her, it was an effective means of managing her distress. Clearly, many other changes had occurred in the 2 years between the introduction of the technique and the follow-up interview but, as reported by Ms. Groth, the technique was a central part of learning to manage her distress.

Ms. Duncan

Ms. Duncan is an older woman who provided care to her husband for around 10 years. In a sense, she always had been a caregiver to her husband because he was a long-standing alcoholic and, prior to his acquiring Korsakoff's syndrome, she had been a helper to him. Once he began to experience small strokes and exhibit signs of dementia, however, her helper role was heightened. She then found it imperative to keep him away from alcohol and also to provide the constant supervision he required.

Mr. Duncan was not an easy person for whom to provide care. He frequently became agitated and often refused to cooperate with Ms. Duncan when she was trying to help him with his personal care tasks. She found herself adapting her life on a daily basis so that her husband would not become agitated. For example, he would hover over her and become very nervous when she was talking to someone on the telephone. Therefore, Ms. Duncan tried to make her telephone conversations as short as possible.

Adapting to her husband's condition was very difficult, especially since Ms. Duncan had a daughter and several grandchildren who lived out of the area. The only way she could keep in touch with them was over the telephone. When her daughter had a new baby, Ms. Duncan had to plan months in advance in order to arrange a visit and make sure that her husband could tolerate the road trip. This became increasingly difficult as he deteriorated further and, eventually, she had to ask her son who lived nearby to stay with him. She was never without worry, however, and always was fearful of him wandering away from the house, which he did on several occasions. Her distress seemed to be constant and seemed to increase as her husband's dementia symptoms worsened.

Ms. Duncan tried several different types of formal supports. The most effective seemed to be a local adult day care center where he went for a few days per week. She found in-home care to be ineffective. Her husband was resistant to care and having someone with whom he was not familiar trying to help him was intolerable; he seemed to become that much more agitated and difficult to deal with. Ms. Duncan tried out several different providers and, during one period a male home health aide seemed to be a good match; however, when he had to discontinue his help, Mr. Duncan was unable to adjust to any of the other providers.

Ms. Duncan found support for herself in many ways, but primarily through the use of support groups. She had attended Al-Anon for many years, and thus was very comfortable with this format. She became part of several on-going caregiver support groups and collected a group of friends through the groups with whom she stayed in regular contact.

Ms. Duncan was interested in learning about the Stress Reduction Technique and was curious about anything that could help her manage her distress level. She met the criteria when she was screened and also reported feeling distressed. As she was taught the various methods, she exhibited enthusiasm about trying them out. She also had a lot to talk about during the sessions, however, and it often was difficult to get her to focus on the actual technique. This was complicated by the fact that the sessions were held in her home where her husband also was present, and often he would wander into the room and she would have to attend to him.

She found most of the techniques helpful; especially, the relaxation techniques during which she inevitably fell asleep while practicing with the instructor. The thought restructuring seemed a little more difficult for her to grasp, and she frequently reported that she was too busy to try out various methods for changing her negative thoughts to positive ones. But, she repeatedly voiced how helpful it was for her to meet with the instructor on a weekly basis and to hear about ways to reduce her distress.

A follow-up interview was conducted approximately 2 years following the sessions. Ms. Duncan reported that her husband recently had been placed in a locked Alzheimer's unit, and that there were repeated problems with his compliance. She said that she had found it increasingly difficult to manage him at home and, since in-home care was not an option, she was left with no choice other than to place him. She said that she was not as tearful as she had been while caring for him at home, but that she had been very frustrated with the details of the placement and consumed with trying to make it work. Ms. Duncan indicated that she felt she was better off because of caregiving, although she was unable to recognize this when she was in the thick of caring for her husband at home, and could only see this now that she could look back over it all.

In looking back over the effectiveness of the Stress Reduction Technique, she responded that it gave her good food for thought, but that she was unable to remember the details. When reminded of the various techniques, she reported that the relaxation technique was helpful and she had continued to utilize this every once in a while. She reported that, although she had been unable to maintain the scheduling of relaxing events, she recently had been able to do this since her husband had been placed. Overall,

Ms. Duncan seemed to indicate that just having someone she could talk to one-on-one on a weekly basis was helpful to her.

Ms. Duncan is an example of a caregiver who felt the process was helpful, but had difficulty identifying how the techniques helped; she could not recall all of the details associated with the methods. It seemed to play some part in her ability to manage the distress related to her caregiving, but it was not clear exactly what part it played.

☐ Summary

As has been demonstrated by the brief review of the caregiver intervention literature, the outcomes from the study performed by Knight, Lutzky, and Olshevski, and the two case examples, the Stress Reduction Technique can be an effective means of helping caregivers cope with their distress. Several factors are important to consider in ensuring that this technique is effective, however. First, it is clear that caregivers should first be assessed to make sure they are experiencing distress and are good candidates for the method. This technique should be targeted to caregivers who demonstrate a need for reducing their distress. Second, caregivers most likely will need assistance from the professional in making sure the techniques are understood, utilized, and helpful. Third, caregivers should be assessed at periodic times following the conclusion of the sessions to evaluate if the techniques have been helpful and to provide any needed follow up.

☐ References

Bourgeois, M., Shulz, R., & Burgio, L. (1996). Interventions for caregivers of patients with Alzheimer's disease: A review and analysis of content, process, and outcomes. *International Journal of Aging and Human Development, 43*, 35–92.

Folkman, S., & Lazarus, R. S. (1988). *Manual for the Ways of Coping Questionnaire*. Palo Alto, CA: Consulting Psychologists Press.

Gallagher, D. E. (1985). Intervention strategies to assist caregivers of frail elders: Current research status and future research directions. *Annual Review of Gerontology and Geriatrics, 5*, 249–282.

Greene, V. L., & Monahan, D. J. (1989). The effect of a support and education program on stress and burden among family caregivers to frail elderly persons. *The Gerontologist, 29*, 472–477.

Knight, B. G., Lutzky, S. M., & Macofsky-Urban, F. (1993). A meta-analytic review of interventions for caregiver distress: Recommendations for future research. *The Gerontologist, 33*, 240–248.

Lovett, S., & Gallagher, D. (1988). Psychoeducational interventions for family caregivers: Preliminary efficacy data. *Behavior Therapy, 19*, 321–330.

Rodin, J., & Salovey, P. (1989). Health psychology. *Annual Review of Psychology, 40*, 533–579.

Toseland, R. W., & Rossiter, C. M. (1989). Group interventions to support family caregivers: A review and analysis. *The Gerontologist, 29*, 438–448.

Toseland, R. W., & Smith, G. C. (1990). Effectiveness of individual counseling by professional and peer helpers for family caregivers of the elderly. *Psychology and Aging, 5*, 256–263.

Zarit, S. H. (1991). Interventions with frail elders and their families: Are they effective and why? In M. A. P. Stephens, J. H. Crowther, S. E. Hobfoll, & D. L. Tennenbaum (Eds.), *Stress and coping in later-life families.* New York: Hemisphere.

Zarit, S. H., Orr, N., & Zarit, J. (1985). *Hidden victims: Caregivers under stress.* New York: New York University Press.

Zarit, S. H., Reever, K. E., & Bach-Peterson, J. (1980). Relatives of the impaired elderly: Correlates of feelings of burden. *The Gerontologist, 20*, 649–655.

CHAPTER

The Context of Stress Reduction: Community Services and Resources for Caregivers

This chapter is an overview of information that caregivers and their helpers should be aware of in order to effectively carry out stress reduction. It is important to understand the social context of older adults and something about case management in order to work with this population. Finding and receiving respite care—regular time off from giving care—will be discussed. In addition, a brief definition of the different types of respite services and community-based care will be covered. The California Statewide System of Caregiver Resource Centers model, which is recognized as a model program, will be used so that the context of this method can be understood and utilized. Next, the importance of planning ahead by engaging in legal and financial planning will be discussed. Last, additional counseling referrals for people who still need help at the end of the stress reduction program will be included.

☐ Respite Services and Community-Based Services

Respite care emphasizes meeting the mental and physical health care needs of the caregiver and care recipient. Respite care comes in many forms, settings and duration. In 1984, California enacted landmark legislation to replicate the model caregiver support program developed by the San Francisco-based Family Caregiver Alliance. The program addresses the emotional, financial, and care providing concerns of the caregiver.

California's Department of Mental Health was required to establish a statewide system of Caregiver Resource Centers (CRCs), modeled after the Family Caregiver Alliance. The CRCs provide a multitude of services to help caregivers, from early intervention to assistance through the various stages of care. The hallmarks of the CRC respite program are flexibility, choice, and consumer control. CRC respite services are provided through the flexible and creative use of local resources, including (but not limited to) in-home care, adult day care services, group care, temporary placement in a facility, and transportation.

Respite care as defined in the CRC's enabling legislation is "Substitute care or supervision in support of the caregiver for the purposes of providing relief from the stresses of constant care provision and so as to enable the caregiver to pursue a normal routine and responsibilities" (Friss-Feinberg, & Kelly, 1995, p. 701). Respite programs such as adult day care, in-home care, and short-term residential placements have the potential to relieve some of the stress on caregivers. Some studies (Gallagher-Thompson, 1994, Knight, Lutzky, & Macofsky-Urban, 1993) have shown that caregivers who have formal help and respite care are better adjusted than those who do not have outside help. It often is difficult to assess the definite impact of community-based services on stress levels of caregivers, because caregivers typically do not access this type of help until late in the course of caregiving when they may be exhausted.

Assistance from social service agencies, when informal support systems are not available from family and friends, can make a caregiver's task a lot easier. Many people have mixed feelings about seeking and receiving outside help. Even though caregivers know they must have help, they may feel that outsiders will not do the job as well as themselves, or that the person they are caring for may be upset by the change. The cost of outside help also is a concern to most people.

> Ms. K, a 65-year-old White woman, was caring for her husband of 44 years and was very distressed. She felt like she did not have any time for herself and did not want to ask her friends or family for assistance in caregiving. She did not want to hire outside help because no one could care for her husband like she did and she did not feel as though she could afford the luxury.

By far, the services most often requested by caregivers are for someone to come into the home and relieve them or to provide housekeeping services. Caregivers can hire their own help or there are a variety of home health agencies in almost every community that can provide a wide range of services, including physical, speech and occupational therapy, nursing care, home health aides, homemakers, and respite care. These agencies vary in the cost per hour of service, the minimum number of hours required, and the particular services provided. It would be beneficial for caregivers to contact a few and compare each to their specific needs.

> It was suggested to Ms. K that there were many services she could try. She had mentioned that there was a local high school down the street, where they had a friendly visitor program. She thought she might call and request a male high school student to come over while she remained at home. By starting slowly, she could see what her own comfort level was with the student as well as her husband's comfort level.

When contacting an agency, it is important for caregivers to have the following information available:

1. The type of service you are seeking. Be as specific as possible.
2. Information about the special needs or problems of the care recipient.
3. Your method of payment.

In order to get the services they need, caregivers may have to make quite a few phone calls and speak with several different people. Here are some tips for caregivers that can help make the process a little easier:

- Write down the name of the person you speak to, in case you need to reach them again.
- Be persistent; polite, but firm.
- You may need to explain your problem more than once; try not to lose your temper and hang up.
- If you are not sure where to start, call your Area Agency on Aging, or 24-hour information and referral service in your area for guidance.

> Ms. K did call the friendly visitor program, but felt like she was getting the runaround. They told her they did not have any male visitors at the present time and were not sure when they might have one available. Ms. K was encouraged to call other programs, and someone she talked to at a local senior center happened to know of a young man who was looking for an after-school job. Ms. K and her husband agreed to meet Sam and see if he would be compatible. After a few visits, Ms. K went for a walk around the block. When she returned, her husband and Sam were engaged in a checker game and appeared to be doing fine together. Ms. K reported that she may try to go for a longer period of time, next week.

Various respite options that offer a range of services are available in most communities. These include in-home respite, homemaker and home health aide services, home-delivered meals, transportation and escort services, chore workers, friendly visitor programs, adult day care programs, overnight out-of-home respite programs, and short-term and overnight respite in a facility.

In-Home Respite

Generally, in-home respite is available 7 days a week, 24 hours a day, and may be scheduled in any way desired by the caregiver. The cost per hour of service varies, depending on whether caregivers find their own helper or whether they hire someone through an agency.

Visiting Nurse Associations and Home Health Agencies

Visiting nurse associations and home health agencies send professional nurses and therapists into the home to provide specific care, including skilled nursing care, physical therapy, occupational therapy, speech therapy, and medical social services. The service must be ordered by a physician in order to qualify for Medicare reimbursement.

Homemaker Services

Homemakers primarily assist with day-to-day household chores. The services provided may include changing beds, doing shopping, and doing light housework. It is important that caregivers interview and select their aide carefully. They should find out about the homemaker's experience and ask for references. They also should inform the homemaker about the physical and mental condition of the care recipient and the services that will be needed. It is important that the homemaker and the care recipient are comfortable with each other. Homemakers sometimes are available to low-income families on a limited basis.

Friendly Visitor Program

Friendly visitors often are students or retirees who come to visit on a regular basis to talk and spend time with homebound older people.

Home-Delivered Meals

Home-delivered meals programs, such as Meals-on-Wheels, deliver a hot, well-balanced lunch and, sometimes, a cold evening meal directly to the home, usually at a reduced cost.

Home Modification

This approach assesses the home setting and develops specific recommendations for environmental modifications. Although little empirical research has been reported on this type of assistance which documents the success of these modifications on reducing troublesome patient behaviors, it seems evident that this type of basic intervention cannot help but improve daily living for caregivers (Pynoos, 1995).

Adult Day Care Respite

Adult day care centers offer part-time respite care. Most offer services on a daily basis, but not overnight or weekend care. There are four types of adult day care centers:

1. Social adult day care. These centers offer social activities and recreational programs. They provide a supervised environment with opportunities to meet new friends and participate in group activities. While most adult day care centers will accept people with Alzheimer's disease, they usually will not accept individuals who are incontinent, wander, or behave in aggressive ways. Staffing will vary according to the needs of each program. Fees will vary but Medicare, Medicaid (Medi-Cal in California), and private insurance typically are not accepted.
2. Alzheimer's day care centers. These centers are special social day care centers that serve people in the moderate to severe stages of Alzheimer's disease or other related dementias. These centers are able to manage participants who are incontinent or who exhibit other problem behaviors.
3. Adult day health care. These centers specialize in providing medical, rehabilitative, and social services for adults over age 18 who have physical or mental impairments. Staff will include nurses and a variety of professional therapists and medical consultants. Fees vary, but Medicare, Medicaid or Medi-Cal, and private insurance typically are accepted.
4. Adult day treatment. These centers specialize in psychological treatment as well as social and recreational activities. Staff will include nurses, social workers, and mental health professionals. Fees vary, but Medicare, Medicaid or Medi-Cal, and private insurance usually are accepted.

It is important to shop around when looking for an adult day care center. Some centers will not accept people with Alzheimer's disease. It is important to question the staff about stipulations concerning wandering, incontinence, and memory impairment. Selecting the best place means asking many questions and visiting the various centers. Most centers encourage caregivers to bring the participant for a visit. Before setting up a visit, caregivers may want to ask the following questions:

- What are the days and hours?
- What is the cost? Is there a sliding scale fee? Are there scholarships available?

- Is transportation available?
- Are there meals or snacks?
- How many participants attend?
- What languages are spoken?
- Does the center serve people with Alzheimer's or other related dementias?
- Is the staff experienced in working with people like my relative?
- Does the staff have any specialized training?
- Can people who wander be safely supervised?

During the visit, caregivers may want to see how the staff members interact with the participants. Ask for, and review, any written material about the center and its policies, activities, menus, and other schedules. Most day care staff will want involvement of caregivers and will answer all their questions and concerns.

Attending an adult day care center can be frightening to the person with dementia as well as to the caregiver. Oftentimes, people do not know what to expect from an adult day care, or they have preconceived notions of what it will be like. It is important for the care recipient to attend regularly and for the caregiver to offer reassurance to the care recipient to make the transition easier. Often, participation in adult day care may become the high point of the week for both the caregiver and the care recipient.

Overnight Out-of-Home Respite Programs

Overnight respite services for caregivers can occur in a variety of settings. Most overnight respite programs provide care to the care recipient for a night, a weekend, or longer. Some of the facilities are traditional care settings, such as a residential care facility or a skilled nursing home, while other programs for care recipients are offered in a "camp" facility. Some programs focus on taking the caregiver, rather than the care recipient, out of the home temporarily for a rest while 24-hour care is provided in the home.

Short-Term, Overnight Respite in a Facility

This option is for caregivers who want relief from the day in and day out duties of caregiving. Relief is available from as little as 24 hours to several weeks. "Reasons expressed by caregivers for this service include need for rest (sleep), or relief, attending family events away from the area, or recuperating from surgery or illness" (Friss-Feinberg, & Kelly, 1995, p. 704). In order to qualify, care recipients must be ambulatory and without severe behavioral problems.

Community-based care is very useful when a caregiver is trying to keep the care recipient in their own home. There may come a time when this will not be possible and 24-hour care in a facility will be necessary.

Senior Centers

Senior centers offer a wide range of activities, social interactions, physical activities, therapy, crafts, congregate meals, legal services, preventive health care, and transportation services. They also may be a valuable source of information for available resources needed to provide respite care.

Case Management Services

Case management is a widely used service that involves assessment, information, and referral data and coordination of services. It serves to cut down the fragmentation of community-based services. Case management is especially useful when a caregiver lives a far distance from the care recipient. Research data appears to be mixed with regard to the efficacy of case management for prevention of long-term institutionalization, but there are results of controlled studies which are positive in that caregivers have used this service heavily when it has been available and have strongly endorsed this model (Gallagher-Thompson, 1994).

☐ Placement in 24-Hour Care

"Although families often go to great lengths to keep aged loved ones at home, they may not be able to provide the best physical and emotional care without experiencing undue stress. When home care and community services are no longer adequate, a person must decide on the best alternative arrangement for meeting personal and health care needs" (*NIA Age Page*, 1996). Placement in a facility depends on the level of care necessary, the functional capacity of the older person, and the amount of behavioral disturbance exhibited. The four types of facilities listed below are in order of the amount of nursing supervision provided, functional capacity of the residents, and cost per month.

Residential Care Facility

Residential care facilities (RCFs) are for individuals who are unable to live alone but do not warrant skilled nursing services. RCFs provide room and board, including special diets of a nontechnical nature, housekeeping, assistance with personal hygiene and grooming, and bedside care during periods of minor or temporary illness. The resident, in general, must be fairly independent. RCFs also provide some recreational and social activities. Some RCFs specialize in care of older people, people with mental disabilities, or people with developmental disabilities. It is suggested that caregivers check out each facility and talk with the owners. RCFs usually are the lowest in cost per month.

Assisted Living

Assisted living facilities accept individuals who are relatively independent but who need assistance with bathing, dressing, getting out of bed, and so forth. These facilities provide some nursing care but do not offer continual nursing services or supervision. Because they provide lower amounts of skilled nursing services, assisted living facilities usually are lower in cost than skilled nursing facilities (SNFs).

Skilled Nursing Facility

SNFs provide continuous nursing services under a registered nurse or licensed vocational nurse. Assistance with activities of daily living (walking, bathing, getting dressed, eating) also are provided. SNFs are required by law to provide recreational activities for the residents. Some SNFs have different levels of care within their facility. Many of these facilities have dementia care units with specially trained staff and accomodations for a person with dementia. Placing a family member in a nursing home can be a difficult decision to make and it often takes time. Many times, families have tried everything else first. Caregivers frequently meet with family resistance and guilt. However, a time may come in the process of caring for a person with dementia when nursing home placement becomes the most responsible decision that a family can make. Going to live in a nursing home is a major change for the frail older person. Their ability to respond to this change will be influenced by how ill they are. Caregivers will want to help them participate in this move and adjust to this change as much as they are able.

When caregivers meet with nursing home administrators, they should discuss financial arrangements in detail and not take anything for granted. If there are things they do not understand, they should not hesitate to ask. All financial agreements should be in writing and caregivers should have a copy of the final arrangements.

It is important to note that the caregiving experience does not stop here. In fact, burden may not decrease . Studies have shown that after placement caregivers often feel even more burdened (Zarit, 1996; Zarit & Whitlatch, 1992; Aneshensel, Pearlin, Mullan, Zarit, & Whitlatch, 1995). Caregivers may feel like they have to be at the facility every day or, if they are not at the facility, they feel guilty or are concerned that their loved one is not being cared for properly.

Psychiatric Locked Facilities

These facilities provide 24-hour nursing services for people with problems such as wandering or violent, disruptive behavior. Unlike SNFs, locked facilities have doors that lock from the inside and walking areas that are secured.

Using respite services and community-based care or placement in a 24-hour care facility may help to reduce some of the distress a caregiver may be feeling, but it is not guaranteed to reduce stress if it is the only strategy used. It is important to combine as many strategies as possible.

Again, it is very helpful if a caregiver can visit several facilities and, if possible, involve the care recipient in selecting one that is the most acceptable. What should caregivers look for and ask when visiting a long-term care facility? Here are some of the things they will want to know:

- Do most of the residents seem reasonably happy and clean?
- Can specific needs, such as diet or physical therapy, be provided?
- What activities and services are available for the residents? Are they encouraged to participate?
- What are the qualifications of the staff?
- How long has the administrator or director of nursing been at the facility?
- What part of the stay will be paid for by Medicare, Medicaid, or private insurance? How much will the resident pay directly?
- You have the right to ask about past or present health department violations.... Ask!

Often, finding the right facility may be difficult. Frequently, the best facilities have long waiting lists or have no vacancies when a caregiver needs it. It would be advantageous for caregivers to begin looking for a suitable facility in advance of when they think they might need it. Names of facilities can be obtained from doctors, clergy, local hospital discharge planners, friends, support group members, local senior centers, or other information and referral services. As mentioned above, it is important to plan ahead. Another area where it is important to plan is the legal and financial aspect of caregiving. The following section will provide more specifics about the legal and financial planning aspect of taking care of a person with dementia.

☐ Legal Alternatives

Managing finances, paying bills, signing contracts, and even the ability to properly understand what ownership means become progressively more difficult for a person with dementia. Often, people simply will give away savings or other assets. In addition, there may be less and less ability to make proper health care decisions.

Depending on the particular situation, there are certain steps or legal alternatives that can be taken to prevent problems in the future. Of course, while some of these steps can be taken without the aid of a lawyer, it may be beneficial in some situations to seek legal advice. The information given here is not to be considered as legal advice.

Generally, there are two categories of systems for legal alternatives. First, for those who plan ahead there are: (a) power of attorney, (b) durable power of attorney, (c) durable power of attorney for health care, and the (d) living trust. Second, for those who do not plan ahead there is conservatorship.

Power of Attorney

The power of attorney gives the caregiver, or whomever is so designated by the individual, the authority to act legally on his or her behalf concerning financial matters. This person is named the attorney-in-fact. The individual may specify either broad areas or very limited areas in which the attorney-in-fact may act on his or her behalf. The power of attorney may be revoked at any time.

The power of attorney is really only valid in the early stages of Alzheimer's disease while the individual is still competent.

Durable Power of Attorney

The durable power of attorney (DPA) is very similar to the power of attorney. It does, however, remain in effect even after the individual is no longer considered competent. In fact, the DPA may contain instructions on when a person is considered incompetent and, therefore, when the DPA will go into effect. This document, often called a springing DPA, may go into effect, for example, only if the individual becomes incapacitated. This may be determined, for instance, when two or more people, such as family members or a physician, state in writing that the person has lost mental capacity. This allows the DPA to go into effect without the oftentimes humiliating court process of determining incompetence. The DPA must be signed while the individual is still competent.

The document itself is fairly simple and is inexpensive to create, but careful thought is necessary when choosing the appointed holder of the DPA. The DPA allows the holder to sign checks, to pay bills or buy necessities, or to sign a contract, for instance, for nursing home care if needed. Gifts can be made by the holder. Often, this may be done to protect the individual's family in an emergency. If the individual develops a tendency to give property away to strangers, the holder can take the property out of the person's hands by putting it into a living trust (discussed below).

Coholders may be appointed. This means that two or more people will act together to manage the individual's assets. This may be used as a safeguard against misconduct by the appointed holders. In contrast to a conservatorship, the holder of the DPA is not under strict court supervision to account for all transactions and, therefore, is subject to mismanagement.

The DPA has been criticized because its acceptance is not mandatory. Some institutions may be unfamiliar with the DPA or suspicious of it and, therefore, may choose not to accept it. This decision would be within their legal rights.

Another potential drawback of the DPA is that, if it becomes necessary to place the individual in an SNF, the holder is not authorized to do so without voluntary consent of the individual. This may be a problem if the individual has become unmanageable at home.

Durable Power of Attorney for Health Care

The DPA for health care authorizes an individual or individuals to make medical decisions for a person if the person is incapacitated and cannot make these decisions. The holder can make the decisions to stop the use of life support machines, to consent to surgical or other medical interventions, or to refuse or terminate treatment. The holder also can decide on donation of the brain after death. He or she is allowed access to medical records and may make them available to others.

The DPA for health care is effective for 7 years from the date signed, unless the document specifies a shorter time period or the person remains unable to make decisions for himself or herself. The DPA for health care remains in effect until the person is able to make his or her own decisions.

The document must be witnessed either by a notary or by two persons, one of whom is not related to the person who has an impairment and is not an heir to that person. The document may not be witnessed by the person granted power of attorney, any health care provider or employee, or any community facility director or employee. The DPA for health care may not be held by the treating health care provider or community care facility or their employees, unless they are related to the patient.

In addition, the holder may not consent to sterilization, psychosurgery, shock treatment, or mental health treatment including outpatient care or commitment to a mental health facility.

The same individual may act as holder of both the DPA for property and the DPA for health care. Both of these powers of attorney may be included in a single document.

The Living Will

The living will is related to the DPA for health care. It is a directive to a person's physician indicating that he or she does not want to be kept alive by artificial means. The living will also allows individuals to appoint someone they trust to make medical decisions for them by including a DPA for health care.

The Living Trust

The living trust appoints a trustee to hold the title to an individual's assets. He or she is obligated to manage these assets according to the terms of the trust. The trust is revocable while the individual is alive, so changes can be easily enforced. At death, the living trust becomes irrevocable and will govern how the trust property is dealt with. Married couples often make a single revocable trust designating themselves as cotrustees. Then, if a patient is deemed incompetent, the healthy spouse acts as sole trustee.

There are many laws governing trusts and the duties of the trustees. There also are wide-ranging legal, financial, and tax implications that may be very complicated. Therefore, good legal advice should be sought when setting up a living trust.

Similar to the DPA, the living trust is less expensive than a conservatorship. For one thing, the trustee does not have to make annual accountings to the court and thus does not need to annually spend money on attorney's fees. Also, if appropriately composed, the living trust for a husband and wife can save a large proportion of the costs of probate. It also can be an excellent tax planning tool.

Conversely, because legal assistance is needed, the living trust itself may be expensive to establish—costing between $750 and $1,000. Also, when the trust becomes irrevocable, there generally will be an immediate tax cost to the estate.

While the living trust probably would deter misuse of the person's assets more efficiently than the DPA, its tighter limitations may make some situations more difficult. The trustee may use assets only for what is stipulated in the trust document. With the DPA, the assets may be used for whatever purpose seems best under the circumstances.

Finally, like the DPA, the living trust does not allow for involuntary placement in an institution.

☐ Options after Incapacity

Guardianship or Conservatorship

A conservatorship may be created through a petition requesting a hearing from the court at which time the conservator of the patient will be appointed. At the hearing, the judge will give the petitioner an opportunity to explain the situation and to discuss requests. Close family members will be notified of the hearing so that they may attend to support or oppose the petition. More than one person may be appointed as coconservators.

There are two types of conservatorships in many states. A person's legal needs will determine which one is appropriate. The first type of conservatorship falls under probate law. Within this category, there are two varieties. First, there is conservatorship of the person. This type of conservatorship is used when a person is no longer able to satisfactorily take care of his or her personal needs, such as health needs, food, clothing, or shelter. Conservatorship of the person also is an option if a person becomes unmanageable and must be placed in a nursing home. Thereafter, should the person demand to be released, the nursing home can legally keep him or her in that protective setting. If this type of conservatorship has not been assigned prior to a placement, a nursing home cannot legally detain a person if he or she wishes to leave.

The second form of probate conservatorship is a conservatorship of the estate. If a person is shown to be unable to manage his or her own finances or to resist fraud or undue influence, this type of conservatorship may be appropriate.

With the conservatorship of the estate, it is possible to divide the community property of a person and his or her healthy spouse into equal shares. This can protect one half of the community property from the financial drain that many husbands and wives experience when they have to place their spouse in a nursing home. Conservatorship also can be used to make a gift of the home to the person's spouse. In this instance, the person no longer has the legal capacity to make gifts to anyone, or to enter into legal contracts.

The same person may be appointed as conservator of the estate and conservator of the person. The central duties of the conservator are to preserve the person's assets. The conservator is responsible for making an accounting of how he or she has managed the person's finances after the first year, and every 2 years following. A conservator must ask the court to approve all expenditures made. The conservator also may ask to be paid for his or her services and be reimbursed for any money advanced for the patient. An attorney is needed to carry out the accounting as well as to implement the conservatorship. As a result, this legal alternative may be expensive. The proper price range for a simple, uncontested conservatorship is between $1,000 and $5,000.

The second type of conservatorship is called the psychiatric conservatorship. This is a more specialized and more limited form of conservatorship than the probate conservatorship. The psychiatric conservatorship permits involuntary commitment to a psychiatric institution for treatment if the individual is harmful to himself or herself or to others or unable to take care of the basic needs of food, shelter, and clothing by reason of a mental disorder.

Involuntary commitment can be ordered by a court only after a full hearing that contains several procedural safeguards. A separate portion of the psychiatric laws provides for involuntary commitment without judicial safeguards for short periods for purposes of emergency treatment and psychiatric evaluation. However, in most states, this temporary commitment must be followed by proper and thorough judicial procedures before long-term involuntary commitment can be ordered.

The question of how to pay for long-term care is a concern for many people. Unfortunately, there are few options. A person can use personal savings, buy long-term care insurance, or, if eligible, apply for Medicaid or Medi-Cal.

☐ Medicaid and Medi-Cal

Medicaid (Medi-Cal in California) is a joint federal and state program that covers the costs of long-term nursing home care for older adults and adults with disabilities, and, in some cases, in-home care (long-term care Medicaid). Coverage varies from state to state. It may cover care in a nursing home, provided the nursing home accepts Medicaid reimbursment. It also can help pay for many of the medical services not covered by Medicare. In some states, it provides medical care for impoverished people (community-based Medicaid). Its purpose is to provide medical care to persons who are in need and do not have sufficient insurance or funds to pay for such care or to provide for those whose medical expenses exceed their income.

Every state establishes its own eligibility standards and administers its own program. Eligibility is based on income and assets. Since every state has different eligiblity requirements, we cannot offer exact figures but can provide an overview; caregivers can refer to state offices for details. A lawyer who is familiar with Medicaid law should be consulted if a person has specific questions about the estate and so forth.

Long-Term Medicaid

Applicants must meet both income asset requirements. There are income limits, and two basic models are used by states. In 20 states, the income eligiblity cutoff is set as a multiple of the state's poverty standard; in 1997, the limit was $1,452 in most of these states. In 30 states, applicants also are eligible if monthly income is less than the monthly cost of nursing home care. When a person qualifies, monthly income must be used to pay for nursing home care; Medicaid pays the balance. The resident is allowed to keep a small amount for a personal needs allowance. A majority of states set a limit at $2,000 for an individual, but this can range from $1,000 to $4,000. The following are examples of what is not included: a home (if a spouse or child with a disability resides there), an automobile, and life insurance (if below an amount specified by the state). Long-term care must be "medically necessary," and each state has a system for making this determination. The criteria vary, and most states use a combination of medical and functional criteria.

In order to prevent the "healthy" spouse from impoverishment, states provide certain protections for income and assets. The rules vary from state to state so it is useful to consult with an attorney. In general, the spouse at home is entitled to keep a monthly maintenance needs allowance (the 1997 federal guidelines were $1,295.00 to $1,975.50). The community spouse also is entitled to keep a portion of the liquid assets. The spousal resource allowance in the 1997 federal guidelines was $15,804 to $79,020. The amount allocated to the spouse in the nursing home must be spent down to the asset level set by the state. The states may deny Medicaid to people who have transferred any asset, including a home, for less than fair market value within 36 months before applying for assistance (look-back period). Anyone needing nursing home care should consult with an attorney before considering asset transfers.

Under certain circumstances, the federal government requires states to try to collect money from the recipient's estate as a way to recoup costs. This is done after determination, through a fair hearing process, that the individual cannot return home and that no one protected under recovery law (spouse, a child who is disabled or a dependent child, certain siblings) is living in the house. The state can seek recovery after a person's death from property other than a house. Estate recovery laws are complex and, again, it is important to consult with an attorney.

Many states have home- and community-based waivers to avoid institutionalizing people in nursing homes when home-based care is a reasonable alternative. Services can include case management; homemaker services; home health aides; personal care services; and adult day health, rehabilitation, and respite care. Not every state offers this, and programs differ from state to state. Programs often have wait lists and are limited in scope.

For more information on legal and financial alternatives, see:

> *Family Survival Handbook: A Guide to the Financial, Legal and Social Problems of Brain-Damaged Adults* by J. Bosshardt, D. Gibson, and M. Snyder. Available through the Family Caregiver Alliance for Brain-Damaged Adults, Inc., 425 Bush Street, Suite 500, San Francisco, CA 94108. Telephone (800) 445-8106.

Many times, finding and utilizing community resources, attempting to get financial and legal affairs in order, and understanding all of the programs available can be stressful. If a caregiver is feeling the need for emotional support, psychosocial interventions also are available .

☐ Psychosocial Interventions

What can caregivers do if they have tried all of the techniques in the book and everything they know to reduce their level of stress, and still feel emotionally and physically exhausted and depleted, or if reducing their level of stress has made them feel better but they still feel like they need help? It then is helpful to explain that sometimes even the most resourceful person needs to seek outside professional help. Some people say they are afraid to ask for professional help because others will think they are "crazy" or "mentally ill." A person does not have to be "crazy" or "mentally ill" to benefit from help. People have many reasons for seeking professional help. Seeking professional help can be a useful and positive way to learn how to reduce one's level of stress. It may mean that:

1. People care enough about themselves to take active steps to reduce their levels of stress.
2. They have developed an awareness of themselves and want to learn how to strengthen their coping skills.
3. They have learned that it is okay to ask for support from others.
4. They care about their family, loved ones, and relationships. They want to be less stressed so that they can be there for their relationships.

Where Can a Person Go For Help?

There are a number of places that a person can go to seek professional help. Some of the possibilities are:

1. Churches or synagogues often have counselors on staff. If they cannot help caregivers, they should be able to refer them to someone who can.
2. Community mental health clinics offer a variety of services. These clinics usually offer various kinds of counseling (individual counseling, family counseling, group counseling, support groups, crisis counseling). Community-based clinics often will see clients for a minimal fee, and many clinics operate with a sliding scale fee schedule where fees are based on income.
3. Universities, colleges, or professional schools often can recommend an appropriate counselor who is in private practice for particular problems. Counselors or therapists in private practice can have varied educations and experiences. They can be social workers, psychologists, marriage and family therapists, or medical doctors. To find a therapist that is appropriate, caregivers can get referrals from professional organizations, health professionals, universities, family members, or friends.

Regardless of where a referral is received, it always is a good idea for caregivers to "interview" the potential counselor, because only caregivers can decide if they will be able to work together with the counselor to gain new skills and a new understanding about their problems.

Questions like, How do I find someone to talk to? What do I look for? Should I go to a group or to individual counseling? and How do I choose someone? often are asked. The most important thing is that the caregiver likes and feels comfortable with the counselor. The caregiver will want to make sure that the professional has experience with dementia and caregiving. Find out where counselors were educated, if they have a degree or specialization in gerontology or aging, what type of approach they use, and the costs of their services. Does insurance cover their services or do they have a payment plan?

Individual Counseling

Individual counseling can help ease the burden and identify positive steps to take, and may assist caregivers in deriving meaning and growth from stressful encounters. Individual psychotherapy has been shown to be effective in helping to manage stress, and is especially important if caregivers are clinically depressed.

Family Meetings

A family meeting can help a family solve a situational problem and provide information to members in order to increase their control over the situation. "Often family meetings are arranged to coordinate and facilitate cooperation among all family members to meet the common goal of caring for the patient" (Bourgeois, Schulz, & Burgio, 1996). In the CRC model, the family meeting usually takes place in one session, but more sessions are available if needed. The meeting should focus on responding to changes occurring in the care recipient or related issues involved in providing care, and should not concentrate on long-standing family conflicts or pathologies. Family meetings can address the tensions and imbalances in the family system created by the care recipient's disabilities (Zarit, Orr, & Zarit, 1985), and also can address the issue of providing more support to the primary caregiver.

Support Groups

A support group may be invaluable to caregivers of people who have memory impairments. Sharing experiences with others who also are trying to cope with a caregiving situation can be both an educational and an encouraging experience.

Caregivers are most likely to receive assistance from a support group than any other type of intervention. Support groups can offer information, emotional support, and the exchange of ideas about managing difficulties. They may assist caregivers in changing their perception of the stressfulness of demands, and help to produce a change in the appraisal of the problem. Membership in a support group may vary. Groups may be specialized for adult children or spouses, or they may be mixed. The group may be led by a professional, or by peers. Some studies (Fitting, Rabins, Lucas, & Eastham, 1986) have demonstrated that male caregivers may have different needs in a support group than female caregivers, and have suggested that perhaps males should be given the opportunity to form their own groups with cofacilitation by a male professional. Studies (Fitting et al., 1986) have shown that male caregivers tend to be more isolated than female caregivers, may be unfamiliar with nontraditional sex role behaviors, and may be uncomfortable with expressing negative feelings.

☐ Summary

The importance of understanding the network of community resources and the options for legal and financial planning cannot be emphasized enough.

Also, in order to avoid the stress related to having to make decisions at times of crisis, it is critical that caregivers plan ahead. This awareness will be useful to caregivers and their helpers in increasing their abilities to carry out stress reduction effectively.

☐ References

Aneshensel, C., Pearlin, L., Mullan, J., Zarit, S., & Whitlatch, C. (1995). *Profiles of Caregiving: The Unexpected Career.* San Diego, CA: Academic Press.

Burgeois, M., Schulz, R., & Burgio, L. (1996). Interventions for caregivers of patients with Alzheimer's disease: A review and analysis of content, process, and outcomes. *International Journal of Aging and Human Development, 43,* 35–92.

Friss-Feinberg, L., & Kelly, K. (1995). A well-deserved break: Respite programs offered by California's Statewide System of Caregiver Resources Centers. *The Gerontologist, 35,* 701–705.

Fitting, M., Rabins, P., Lucas, M., & Eastham, J. (1986). Caregivers for dementia patients: A comparison of husbands and wives. *The Gerontologist, 26,* 248–251.

Gallagher-Thompson, D. (1994). Direct services and interventions for caregivers: A review of extant programs and a look to the future. In M. Cantor (Ed.), *Family caregiving: Agenda for the future* (pp. 102–122). San Francisco: American Society on Aging.

Gonyea, J. (1989). Alzheimer's disease support groups: An analysis of their structure, format and perceived benefits. *Social Work in Health Care, 14,* 61–72.

Kahan, J., Kemp, B., Staples, F., & Brummel-Smith, K. (1985). Decreasing burden in families caring for a relative with a dementing illness: A controlled study. *Journal of the American Geriatric Society, 33,* 664–670.

Knight, B., Lutzky, S., & Macofsky-Urban, F. (1993). A meta-analytic review of interventions for caregiver distress: Recommendations for the future research. *The Gerontologist, 33,* 240–249.

Pynoos, J. (1995). Supportive Services? Fine. But how about supportive surrounding? *Perspective on Aging, 24,* no. 4, 20–23.

Quayhagen, M. P., & Quayhagen, M. (1988). Alzheimer's stress: Coping with the caregiving role. *The Gerontologist, 28,* 391–396.

Zarit, S. (1996). Interventions with family caregivers. In S. Zarite and B. Knight (Eds.), *A Guide to Psychotherapy and Aging* (pp. 139–159). Washington, DC: American Psychological Association.

Zarit, S., Orr, N., & Zarit, J., (1985). *The Hidden Victims of Alzheimer's Disease: Families Under Stress.* New York: New York University Press.

Zarit, S., & Whitlatch, C. (1992). Institutional placement: Phases of the transition. *The Gerontologist, 32,* 665–672.

INDEX

(f, figure; t, table)

Abbreviated progressive relaxation training (ABRT), 52
Acceptance coping, 11
Active coping, 10
Adult day care, 118, 121–122
Affect, relationship to cognition, 82
African American
  caregivers, burden appraisal, 9, 17
  church support network, 22–23
  coping style, 23–25
  cultural tradition, 19–20
  extended family, 19, 20
  family dynamics, 20–21
  health risks of caregivers, 30
  view of illness, 23
Aging, and disease, 1, 2
Al-Anon, support group, 113
Alzheimer's day care centers, 121
Alzheimer's Disease Research Center, ix, x, xii
Anderson, N. B., 18, 26
Anxiety, and cognitive restructuring, 82
Appraisal, of stressfulness, 36
Area Agency on Aging, 119
Assisted living facilities, 124
Avoidance coping, 10, 109

Baseline, for stress, 39
Beck, Aaron T., 67, 82
Behavior problems, impact on caregiver, 6, 7
Brief Symptom Inventory, 106
Burns, D., 83

California Statewide System of Caregiver Resource Centers (CRCs), 117
Cardiovascular disease, and stress, 37
Cardiovascular reactivity (CVR), 18, 29, 106, 109
Caregiver Resource Centers (CRCs), respite services, 118, 134
Caregivers
  definition, 2
  similarities among, 18
Caregiver stress, interventions, 100, 101t–102t
Case example
  African American caregiver, 21–22
  African American niece caregiver to aunt, 56–59
  married daughter caregiver to mother, 91–93
  middle-aged daughter caregiver both parents, 46–48
  middle-aged daughter caregiver to mother, 59–60, 60–62
  middle-aged son caregiver to mother, 43–46
  spouse caregiver to husband, 76–79, 93–96, 109–112, 112–114
Case management services, 123
Catastrophizing, 46
Center for Epidemiological Studies Depression Scale, 106
Church, mutual aid provider to African Americans, 22
Cognition, relationship to affect, 82

Cognitive-behavioral approach to therapy, 81
Cognitive-behavioral modification, 82
Cognitive-behavioral therapy, with depressed caregivers, 84
Cognitive distortion, 83
  of caregiving time, 74
Cognitive redefinition, 25
Cognitive restructuring, x, 9, 11, 81–84
Cognitive Therapy and the Emotional Disorders, 82
Cohabitation, among African Americans, 20, 21
Community-based services, 117–123
Community resources information, xi
Conflict, in support systems, 11
Conservatorship, 129–130
Control, regaining with Relaxing Events Schedule, 69
Coping, definition, 36
Coping styles, 9–11
  of African Americans, 23–25
Counseling, sources of, 133
Creativity, in adapting techniques for caregivers, 96
Cultural mechanisms, for coping with stress, 26
Cultural tradition, African American, 19–20
Cycle of distress, 38, 68
  reversing, 86

Daily planner, 72f
Daily Stress Rating (DSR) form, 35, 40–41, 41f–42f, 74
Daughter, as primary caregiver, 2
Daughter-in-law, as primary caregiver, 2
Decision making shift, Alzheimer caregiver, 77, 94
Decision to place, 12
Deep breathing, in progressive relaxation, 53–54
Dementia caregivers, stress in, 10, 11, 12
Dementia/physically-frail elder caregivers, studies of, 100, 103
Dementing illness education, xi
Depression
  in caregivers, 3, 4, 67
  and cognitive-behavioral therapy, 85
  and cognitive restructuring, 82
  and pleasant activities, 66
  and stress, 37

Diagnostic Interview Schedule (DIS), 3
Dilworth-Anderson, P., 18, 26
Distractions, to relaxation exercise, 53, 58
Distress, reaction to negative stress, 37
Durable power of attorney (DPA), 126–127
  for health care, 127–128

Eldest son, Asian primary caregiver, 3
Eligibility, Medicaid, 131
Ellis, Albert, x, 9, 82
Emotion regulation, coping style, 10
Emotional distress, in caregivers, 3–4
Escape-avoidance coping, 10
Estate recovery laws, 132
Extended family, African American, 3, 19, 20

Family caregivers, 2
Family dynamics, African American, 20–21
Family meetings, 134
Family Survival Handbook: A Guide to the Financial, Legal and Social Problems of Brain-Damaged Adults, 132
Feeling Good: The New Mood Therapy, 83
Female-headed families, African Americans, 20
Fictive kin, African American, 3, 19, 20
Folkman, S., ix, 7, 10, 36
Follow through, Relaxing Events Schedule, 74–76, 78, 79
Frailty, average period of, 2
Friendly visitor programs, 119, 120

Gastrointestinal disorders, and stress, 37
General distress model, 4
Generalized anxiety disorder, and cognitive-behavioral therapy, 85
Global Symptom Index (GSI), 107
Goal setting, in scheduling relaxation, 75
Guardianship, 129–130

Help-seeking caregivers, selection bias, 4
Hidden Victims of Alzheimer's Disease, The: Families Under Stress, x
Home-delivered meals, 120
Home health aides, 118
Homemaker services, 120
Home modification, 120–121
Hooker, K., 4
Housekeeping services, 118

Imaginal relaxation, 52, 53
Immune response, and caregiving, 27
Immune system, impact of stress on, 37
Individual counseling, 100, 101t, 102t, 133
Informal Caregivers Survey, 5
In-home respite, 120
Insomnia
    and ABRT, 52
    cognitive restructuring, 85
    progressive relaxation, 52
Instructions
    progressive relaxation, 54–55
    visualization, 56
Internal dialogue, 81
Irrational beliefs, 83

Jacobson, E., 51

Katz, Anne, x
Kiecolt-Glaser, J., 27, 28, 30

Lazarus, R., ix, 7, 10, 36
Lewinsohn, Peter., x, 4, 39, 66, 67
Life expectancy, increase in, 1
Living trust, 128–129
Living will, 128

Mahoney, M., 83
Major depressive disorder, and
        cognitive-behavioral therapy, 85
Managing stress, 39, 68
McGrath, J. E., 36
Medicaid, 130–131
    long-term, 131–132
Meichenbaum, Donald, x, 4, 9, 82
Memory impairment, impact on caregiver,
    6
Metabolic change, in caregivers, 29
Minorities
    caregivers, 17
    view of illness, 23
Monitoring stress, xi, 39–43, 42f, 43f
Mood, and pleasant activities, 67, 68
Muscle groups, in progressive relaxation,
    52
Mutual concern, among African
    Americans, 19

Never-married, African Americans, 20

Non-relative caregiving, African American,
    19, 21
Nuclear family, White American, 19

Objective health measures, caregiver, 5–6
Older adult, cognitive-behavioral strategies
    with, 85
Older population, increases in, 1
Open-ended questions, 19
Overnight respite services, 122

Pain management, and ABRT, 52
Perceived physical health, of caregiver, 5
Personality factor neuroticism, and
    perceived health, 5, 9
Physically-frail elder/dementia caregivers,
    studies of, 100, 103
Physiological stress, and caregiving,
    27–29
Planning, in developing Relaxing Events
    Schedule, 69
Pleasant activities, and care recipient, 68
Pleasant Events Theory, 65, 68
Positive reappraisal, 25, 29
Power of attorney, 126
Prayer, as African American coping
    resource, 24
Prescreening, caregivers for intervention,
    108
Primary care giver, responsibility of, 2
Problem solving, caregiver's, 67
Problem-solving coping, 10
Problem-solving training, study group, 104,
    105, 108
Progressive relaxation
    case examples of use, 56–59, 59–60,
        60–62
    instructions for, 54–55
    steps in, 53
    term, 51
Psychiatric locked facilities, 125
Psychoeducational group approach x,
    99–100, 101t, 102t
Psychoeducational individual tutoring
    study, 104–109
    participants, 105
    results, 107–108
Psychosocial interventions, meta-analytic
    review of, 101t, 103

Rational emotive therapy (RET), 9, 82
Relaxation training, x, 4
Relaxing events, x, 4
    case examples, 70, 71
    identification of, 70, 71f, 77
    scheduling of, 72–73, 78
Relaxing Events Schedule, 65
    case example, 76–79
    follow through, 74–76
    steps in, 69
Relaxing Events Theory, 68
Religious coping, African American, 24,
    25
Residential care facilities (RCFs),
    123–124
Resistance
    to scheduling of relaxation, 73, 74
Respiratory infection, in caregivers, 28
Respite care, 13
    definition, 118
    meta-analytic review of programs, 102t,
    103
Reward contract, in scheduling relaxation,
    76
Rewards, for self-change, 90
Robert Ellis Simon Foundation, ix
Role strain, adjustment to in long-term
    caregiving, 23
Rubber-band, reminder with worried
    thoughts, 89, 95

Schedule for Affective Disorders and
    Schizophrenia (SADS), 3
Scheduling of relaxing events, x, 72–74
Schulz, R., 5
Self-blame, 10, 109
Self-change, elements of, 90
Self-efficacy, of caregivers, 67
Self-instructional training, 82
Self-monitoring, thoughts, 81
Self-talk, 9, 11, 89
Selye, H., 35
Senior centers, 123
Short Portable Mental Status
    Questionnaire, 20
Short-term residential facilities, 118,
    122–123
Skilled nursing facility (SNF), 58, 96,
    124–125

Skills training intervention, 102t, 104
Social isolation, caregivers, 66
Social learning, model of depression,
    66
Social networks, buffer against stress,
    26–27
Social service agency, tips for contacting,
    119
Social support, 11–12
    definition, 18
    network, African American, 19
Spielberger State-Trait Anxiety Inventory,
    106
Spousal resource allowance, 131
Spouse, as primary caregiver, 2
States of Mind (SOM) model, positive and
    negative cognition, 84
Step-by-step change, 90
"Stop," reminder with worried thoughts,
    89, 96
Stress
    definitions of, 36
    environmental, 36
    as physiological response, 36
    as reaction to change, 36
    as term, 35
Stress and coping theory, 7, 8f
Stress Inoculation Training, 4, 9
Stress Level Monitoring, 38
    case examples of use, 43–46, 46–48
Stress-Neutral Thoughts, 81, 85, 86, 89,
    111
    case examples, 91–93, 93–96
Stress reduction approach, to caregiving
    intervention, x, xi
Stress reduction training, study group, 104,
    105, 108
Stress Reduction Technique, effectiveness
    of, 99, 108–109
Support groups, 100, 101t, 102t, 103,
    134

Thought Tracking Record (TTR), 81,
    87f–88f, 87–89
Time course, caregiving, 7
Tingstad, Hortense, ix
Tingstad Older Adult Counseling Center,
    ix
Tracking stress level, 39, 40

Visiting nurse associations, 120
Visualization
   case examples of use, 56–59, 59–60,
     60–62
   description of technique, 55
   instructions for, 56

Wait list subjects, study group, 104, 105,
   106
"Wear and tear" model, caregiving, 3, 7
White Americans
   nuclear family, 19

view of illness, 23
Worried thoughts, 86–87
   identification of, 88
   managing and decreasing, 89–90
Writing
   commitment to Relaxing Events
     Schedule, 69
   worried thoughts on index card, 89–90,
     92–93

Zarit Burden Interview (ZBI), 105